How to Fight Depression

A Beginner Guide for Overcoming Depression

Howard Patel

How to fight Depression

Copyrights Notice

Limited Liability

Please note that the content of this book is based on personal experience and various information sources.

Although the author has made every effort to present accurate, up-to-date, reliable, and complete information in this book, they make no representations or warranties concerning the accuracy or completeness of the content of this book and specifically disclaim any implied warranties of merchantability or fitness for a particular purpose.

Your particular circumstances may not be suited to the example illustrated in this book; in fact, they likely will not be. You should use the information in this book at your own risk.

All trademarks, service marks, product names, and the characteristics of any names mentioned in this book are considered the property of their respective owners and are used only for reference. No endorsement is implied when we use one of these terms.

This book is only for personal use. Please note the information contained within this document is for educational and entertainment purposes only and no warranties of any kind are declared or implied. Readers acknowledge that the author is not engaged in providing any kind of medical, dietary, nutritional, psychological, psychiatric advice, nor professional medical advice.

Please consult a doctor, before attempting any techniques outlined in this book. Nothing in this book is intended to replace common sense or medical consultation or professional advice and is meant only to inform. By reading this book, the reader agrees that under no circumstances is the author responsible for any losses, direct or indirect, which are incurred as a result of the use of the information contained within this document, including, but not limited to, errors, omissions, or inaccuracies.

Table of Contents

Introduction

Overview of Depression

Depression is America's most common mental health issue. It affects 17 million of all ages, groups, and races each year.

Depression is a serious disease and it needs to be understood by everyone whether you are suffering from depression, have a friend or loved one who is suffering from it, or just hear about it.

Even if you don't have the disease or know someone who's suffering from it, it's still good to get to know it so you can recognize its symptoms at any point in time, get diagnosed immediately, and get the help you or your friend or loved one needs. The early diagnosis of it is the secret to treating and overcoming depression over time. You can beat it easily if you can recognize its symptoms in time and seek treatment.

What is depression?

The usual feeling of poor emotions, sorrow, or feeling down should not be confused for depression. Such feelings are normal reactions to day-to-day events and are often overcome in a short period. If someone is depressed or has mood swings continuously for weeks, months, or longer and it restricts the individual from doing his or her regular activities; that could be depression.

There are various kinds of depression, major depression, dysthymia, adjustment disorder, seasonal affective disorder, and bipolar or manic depression.

Causes of Depression

Depression ranges from genetic causes to major life events. That is, if some family members have had depression, it increases the likelihood of the person getting depression. And if an individual experiences sudden life changes such as losing a loved one or going to a new region, or someone has a heartbreak, the individual may become depressed.

Other feasible causes of certain kinds of depression or diseases could be chronic disease or side effects.

Diagnosing Depression

See a mental health specialist for a thorough clinical assessment for precise treatment. You should have experienced at least 5 of the following signs continuously over at least 2 weeks to qualify for treatment.

Signs and symptoms of Depression

Having little interest or enjoyment in doing stuff, Feeling down, difficulty falling asleep, or sleeping too much, feeling exhausted or having little power, loss of appetite or overeating, Feeling bad about yourself, or that you or your friends have failed to concentrate on stuff going or talking so slowly.

Especially if you find such signs in kids, do not ignore them. Untreated depression can present a life-threatening situation.

Treating Depression

If your doctor suspects depression, then he or she can refer you to a psychiatrist, psychologist, or certified social worker who will then provide you with an adequate diagnosis of depression.

Early identification and diagnosis are the keys to overcoming depression rapidly. Don't stop therapy!

There's nothing to be scared of, more than 80% of poor individuals are effectively handled. A psychiatrist or psychologist can conduct a thorough assessment and initiate a therapy scheme with you that may include counseling, medicine, or both.

Good coping mechanisms and alternative therapies still exist and can be used to alleviate depression symptoms.

SECTION 1

In-depth Understanding of Depression

I think the word "depression" has come to be used very casually and generally. The statements that used to be mere "mood swings," "boredom," "solitude" and "sorrow" have now been blown into "depression."

While individuals have begun to believe that they are suffering from a "psychological disorder," many individuals with severe pathological "depression" are held very lightly and are not supplied with appropriate social support and therapy services. Either way, one of the major concerns is the impact.

WHO states, "Depression can be long-lasting or recurrent, significantly impairing the capacity of an individual to function at the job or college or deal with everyday lives. Depression can contribute to suicide at its most serious stage."

Understanding DEPRESSION in its true context places a moral responsibility on us - NOT USE THE WORD CASUALLY FOR EVERY SADNESS FEELING, GUILT, LOSS, FRUSTRATION, IRRITABILITY ETC.

Here's what the American Psychiatric Association tells us— the death of a loved one, the loss of a career, or the end of a partnership are hard times an individual can overcome.

Development in reaction to such stressful circumstances is common for emotions of sorrow or grief. Yet depression and sadness are not the same things. While sorrow will evade over the moment, depression may remain for months, even years.

It also states— Depression is a severe medical condition that harms how you feel, how you believe, and how you behave.

Depression has a range of signs, but the most frequent is a profound sense of sorrow or a marked loss of concern or fun activity.

Other signs include:

- Appetite changes that lead to weight loss or diet-free benefits.
- Inadequate or excessive sleep.
- Energy loss or enhanced tiredness.
- Unrest or irritability.
- Feelings of improper guilt or worthlessness.
- Hard to think, concentrate, or make choices.
- Death or suicide thoughts or suicide attempts.

Let's know then that EVERY SADNESS is NOT DEPRESSION. In life, none is saved from difficulties and adverse issues. These issues and difficulties are the possibilities that are given to us to fulfill our objective in existence. These difficult moments often show the magnitude of human resilience and make us do stuff that surprises us and others.

Certainly, the times are difficult, but we can feel a little stronger each time we come out of it or when the time changes. With adequate plans, advice, and encouragement, most life problems can be fixed.

It is therefore of utmost significance to recognize people who are threatened with clinical depression from among the bunch that avoids loosely tossing the' D' term around to face the daily difficulties of life. Many need assistance and therapy immediately.

Dimensions of Depression

Depression is an unusually prevalent experience. The Centers for Disease Control (CDC) reports that for some type of depression (e.g., major depression, dysthymic disease) about 1 in 10 teenagers is struggling with depressive diseases that fulfill the diagnostic requirements. Depression-that is how depression manifests and explains what builds it. The causes of depression are often hard to discern from their signs. You have a structure to understand how your depression can impact your lives by looking at the distinct aspects of depression.

Behavioral aspect: Behavioral view holds that depression is the result of poor concentrations of inactivity induced by unfulfilled environmental benefits. Tiredness, absence of pleasure, and bad motive are the primary causes of depression. When responding to your cognitive dimension, we concentrate on enhancing your life's operations by establishing a timetable that involves pleasurable operations to follow.

Cognitive aspect: Depression results from the behavioral view and is preserved by your holding of adverse ideas and opinions.

An extensive depression study informs us that you tend to believe badly about yourself, others, and the future when you're depressed. Cognitive therapists believe thinking leads to emotions and behavioral patterns. In responding to your depression's cognitive dimension, we tackle the adverse ideas and opinions that you retain, for instance, by assisting you to be aware of how you feel and start replacing adverse ideas with more genuine ones. This, in turn, helps improve morale.

Emotional aspect: Emotions are very complicated and the connection between feelings and depression does not have a single view. However, there is proof that informs us about the connection between the two stuff. First, depression may lead to unresolved loss-related sorrow. If we don't grieve the difficulties of life properly — for example, the loss of a job, the death of a friend or pet, a traumatic experience— our grief remains unprocessed and psychologically heavy. There is also a big body of proof that informs us that if we "things" our emotions— that is if we prevent feeling and expressing them— our likelihood of growing depressed. This is why it is so important to be willing to speak about your emotions. When we look at your depression's mental dimension, we bring phrases into your emotions and comprehend them and the significant data they contain in doing so.

Biological aspect: Depression's biological view represents what occurs when you are depressed in the brain and other sections of the body. Depressive signs are associated with low concentrations of certain neurotransmitters such as serotonin, dopamine, and norepinephrine. Physical depression signs, including exhaustion, absence of motive, sleep disruption, and improved or reduced appetite point to depression's biological aspect.

This is where antidepressants can be most useful in reducing these signs as they target neurotransmitter concentrations in the brain.

This is also where practice becomes crucial for people struggling with depression. Several surveys have shown that everyday periodic practice of medium to elevated intensity can be as efficient as some kinds of antidepressants. When we look at this dimension of your depression, we take into account the function of enhanced activity and the chance of referral for medication and dietary advice.

Social aspect: Depression results from and is preserved in your relationship problems from the social view. Interpersonal psychotherapy— a type of depression treatment — focuses specifically on issues such as relationship role changes and communication abilities. When we look at your depression aspect, we assist you to boost your personal touch and enhance your present interactions to make them more satisfying and meaningful.

Existential aspect: human humans are animals in search of meaning. Naturally, we are looking for a broader view to comprehend our issues. Depression may lead to an absence of significance in your lives from the Existential view. When you feel detached from your potential— from what you are called to do with your life— it makes sense to feel depressed and unmotivated, particularly when you know that your time on this planet is restricted. When we look at your depression's existential dimension, we operate to define the discrepancy between how you are living your lives at the moment and how you want to live.

We are working to assist you in articulating your principles and developing a strategy to advance towards them. We're helping you to discover significance.

Last, some intellectuals claim that depression is a question of the soul. Psychologists such as James Hillman and Thomas Moore argue that depression symptoms are a call from the soul to attend to some internal wound, at the core of which are invaluable donations.

When we attend to the depression aspect of the soul, we listen carefully to your signs and pursue them inwardly — as if you pursue a good thread— to figure out what your heart is calling you to do at this moment.

Types of Depression

Depression can exist in many forms. It can last for months or even years before it is identified. Statistics have shown that this year millions of Americans would experience some form of depressive disorder. Sadly, fewer than 1/3 of these people are going to seek help. The sufferers often do not yet realize that they are ill.

Stress is popular every day in the modern world. Navigating the obstacles in life is tougher. Most households live week after week. Economic troubles have made having a good job more complicated than ever. Stress can make you feel depressed.

There are common depression forms. Some of the marks have the same definition. Depressive disorder happens psychologically, socially, professionally, or manically. There is also the fact that it becomes too serious to allude to the disease's final stages. Depressive disorder can result from a variety of causes. Simple biology, brain chemistry issues are some of those. It is also borne by DNA. Those with illness family history are in danger.

Categories:

Major Depression - This is the most serious type, given the number of symptoms and severity of symptoms, but there are significant differences in symptoms and severity among people.

You don't need to feel suicidal to have a major case, and you don't need to have a record of hospitalization either, although some people with major depressive symptoms have both of these reasons.

Dysthymic disorder - That applies to small to moderate levels that last for at least two years and often longer. Although the effects are not as extreme as the original variant, they are more frequent and treatment prone. Through their condition, most patients with dysthymia experience a major case at some stage.

Unspecified - This classification is used to help scientists who are researching certain specific types and do not want to overlap their results with a generic diagnosis. This involves persons with a serious case, but not too extreme to have a major form classification.

It also includes people with recurrent, mild, who was not around long enough for a dysthymic disorder to be identified.

Adjustment Disorder - This class describes what happens in a major life stressor or crisis.

Bipolar - This condition involves high and low mood swings as well as several other severe signs that are not found in other disorder types.

Other Depressive Class Types:

Post-Partum - Major depressive disorder after childbirth. Depressive symptoms usually start within four weeks after giving birth and may differ in duration and intensity.

Seasonal Affective Disorder (SAD) - A form of depressive disorder characterized by major case events that happen at a particular time of year (e.g. autumn, winter). Depressive events have happened at least twice over the past two years without any occurrences happening at a different time.

Anxiety - Not an approved category (as the DSM defines). Anxiety also often happens with anxiety, though. A depressed person may also have symptoms of anxiety (e.g. panic attacks) or an anxiety disorder (e.g. PTSD, panic disorder, social phobia, generalized anxiety disorder) in this situation.

Constant - Major period of depression lasting at least two years.

Double - Someone with dysthymia (chronic mild) and a major depressive disorder (significant depressive symptoms lasting at least two weeks).

Endogenous - Endogenous body sense. For no apparent reason, this category is characterized as feeling depressed.

Situational and reactive (also known as Depressed Mood Adjustment Disorder) - Depressive symptoms that evolve in response to a particularly stressful situation or occurrence (e.g. job loss, end of a relationship). Such symptoms occur within 3 months of the stressor and do not continue more than 6 months after the stressor has stopped (or its consequences). Symptoms of depression cause significant discomfort and affect normal activity (e.g. friendships, employment, school) and do not follow major depressive disorder guidelines.

Agitated - A form of major depressive disorder marked by anxiety such as physical and emotional restlessness, irritability, and insomnia, which is the reverse of many stressed people who have low energy and feel physically and mentally slowed down.

Psychotic - Huge episode of schizophrenia with psychotic symptoms such as visions (e.g. hearing voices), paranoia (false beliefs).

Atypical (Subtype of Major and Dysthymia) - Characterized by a sudden change of attitude in reaction to positive events and two (or more) of the following:

- significant weight gain or rise in appetite
- excessive sleeping
- heavy feeling in arms or legs
- long-standing history of rejection resistance

Melancholic (Subtype of Major Depressive Disorder) - Common symptoms of this type. There are also three (or more) of the following:

- Sad mood with a specific consistency (e.g. separate from feeling depressed while grieving)
- The depressive feeling becomes usually worse in the evening
- Waking up earlier than usual (at the last 2 hours)
- Noticeable irregular activity and slowing down
- Significant decrease in appetite and weight loss
- Irregular and improper feeling

Catatonic (Subtype of Major Depressive Disorder) - This group is characterized by at least two of the following:

- Lack of voluntary activity or failure to respond to one's surroundings
- Excessive motion (without intent and not in reaction to one's environment)

- Strong aversion to instructions/suggestions or incapacity/unwillingness to communicate
- Extraordinary or improper voluntary movement or attitude

For example, the aim of treatment can vary or it may be recommended that specific medications treat those symptoms.

Common factors may contribute to various types. Misuse of drugs may contribute to depressive disorder. It may be practiced by both alcoholics and drug abusers. Historically, a mental disorder is synonymous with a stigma. Some found it a psychological defect before mental illness was accepted as a condition.

As a consequence, medication was not administered in a fashion that could be of benefit to the client. Negative effects continue through all depression levels. Treatment also requires early detection.

Perhaps one of the most common forms of major depressive disorder. You probably know a few people who are suffering from it. The sufferer seems to be riding about on his or her back with the weight of the world. He or she is unwilling to engage in regular activities and seems certain that he or she will always be in this miserable condition. Sexual activity and appetite are low in desire or weight loss.

Atypical: is a slightly different deviation from the usual form. Often joy or feelings of elation can be felt by the sufferer. Atypical form signs include exhaustion, sleeping in, overeating, and gaining weight. People who suffer from it feel their attitude (i.e. performance, affection, and praise) is influenced by outside occurrences. Episodes can last for months or a person can live forever with it.

Psychotic: sufferers begin seeing and seeing images unreal—noises, words, and visions that do not occur. These are also delusions, which are normally more associated with someone who has psychosis. The delusions are not "good" as they are triggered by depression. The sufferer imagines noises and pictures that are disturbing and pessimistic.

Dysthymia: Most individuals are just wandering around seemingly discouraged— either gloomy, dark, and melancholic. They've been all their life like this. This is a dysthymia-a disease that people don't even know about but deal with daily. We feel unimportant, unhappy, afraid and just do not enjoy our lives thru childhood. A form of the drug is helpful to it.

Manic: can be described as an emotional disorder that may sometimes be very quick due to shifting mood shifts. Individuals with manic depressive disorder have an extraordinarily high suicide rate.

Behavioral: what medical professionals term an affective behavioral illness, or SAD, is something that only happens at a certain time of year, typically in winter. It is sometimes labeled "spring blues." It can be very serious even though it is repetitive.

Cyclothymic syndrome: A milder version of bipolar disorder, yet more lasting. The attitude of a patient alternates from a less extreme mania (known as hypomania) to a less severe case.

Mood disorder-induced or precipitated by a known or unknown physical condition such as hypothyroidism.) Drug-Induced Mood Imbalance may be triggered or precipitated by the use or misuse of factors such as opioids, tobacco, hormones, and toxins.

Premenstrual Dysphoric Disorder: This is a rare type of psychological disorder that affects a limited percentage of menstruating women. It is a cyclical syndrome in which every month people may feel depressed and irritable before their menstrual period for one or two weeks.

What is a depressive disorder exactly?

Since the beginning of recorded history, depressive disorders have been with mankind. King David and Job died from this affliction in the Bible. Hippocrates alluded to it as gloomy, or black bile literally.

Black bile was the four senses of humor (fluids) that represented the basic theory of clinical physiology of that period, along with saliva, phlegm, and green bile. It is also labeled psychiatric anxiety, has been depicted for hundreds of years in literature and the arts, but what do we say now when we relate to a depressive disorder? It was seen as an inherent personality deficiency in the 19th century.

Freud attributed the creation of negative emotions with shame and confrontation in the first half of the 20th century. The writer and contemporary sufferer of depressive disorder, John Cheever, wrote of confrontation and encounters with his family as affecting his condition growth.

Symptoms that help a psychiatrist diagnose the condition include:

- persistent feelings of sadness, irritability, and stress
- reduced enthusiasm and enjoyment in usual activities or hobbies
- loss of strength, feeling tired without lack of activity
- increase of appetite, significant weight loss, or weight gain
- a shift in sleep patterns, such as difficulty sleeping, early morning waking, From chronic diseases including heart disease through the perception of pain, age, and sleep.

Sexual problems - sexual desire and sexual performance can be influenced by medications.

Sleep problems - Find out how sleep disruption is induced by this disease and get some useful tips to help sleep problems.

Warning Signs

Once the infection has advanced to a degree too extreme to treat the disease. The applications for help have not been received and the potential to solve the problem is now disappearing. Combine medications or rehabilitation for a treatment that works.

Support groups are also present that can support. For clinical studies, you can also find some natural herbal medicines that have been proven effective. The good news is that medications are accessible that are very successful to support those who are stressed. Only about one-third of those who are suicidal receive treatment, though. This is disappointing since in only a few months, about 80-90% of those seeking treatment rising feel better. Many claims that the consequence of personal weakness and character flaw is depression. That's just not real. Including hypertension, heart disease, or any other illness.

About 80% of all severe cases of anorexia and bulimia have a coexisting clinical diagnosis of depression. Depression is in and of itself a very frustrating and all-consuming illness. Depression, though, is beyond destruction in tandem with an eating disorder and is often hidden within the eating disorder itself.

Depression appears different in eating disorder patients than it does in mood disorder clients alone. Another way to describe how depression occurs in an eating disorder sufferer is secret suffering.

Depression takes on increased quality of misery and self-hatred of eating disorder patients and becomes a manifestation of their personality, not a collection of unpleasant symptoms. Depression is associated with eating disorder signs, and the depressive symptoms are often not distinguishable from the eating disorder due to this interwoven value. The purpose of this book is to explain some of the similarities and variations in how depression is expressed in someone with anorexia or bulimia. One aim is to provide ideas that begin promoting optimism within the counseling environment for these desperate clients.

In coping with instances of an eating disorder, it is important to understand that it is most likely present on two points when major depression is involved. Second, a history of persistent, low-level, dysthymic depression will be apparent, and second, signs will be associated with one or more severe bouts of acute major depressive disorder. The depression's severity and acuteness are not always appeared instantly in how the client expresses their eating disorder. Taking medical histories may show persistent discouragement, feelings of inadequacy, low self-esteem, appetite disruption, sleep disturbance, low energy, exhaustion, attention problems, decision-making difficulties, and a general sense of unhappiness and ambiguous distress.

Since most eating disorder patients have not been seeking treatment for many years, it is not unusual for this form of persistent dysthymic depression to have been from two to eight years of their life somewhere. Clinical records will also show that there is a concomitant record of extreme signs of major depression as the eating disorder intensified or became increasingly serious in its severity. In those with long-standing eating disorders, frequent periods of major depression are often seen.

Simply put, eating disorder patients have long been depressed, they have not felt good about themselves for a long time, they have long felt helpless, and they have experienced violent periods of depression in which life has become much worse and harder for them.

Special characteristics

An extreme and elevated level of self-hatred and self-contempt is one of the most unique features of depression in someone recovering from an eating disorder. This may be because those with such major depressive disorders in combination with an eating disorder have a much more specific negative or identity-based meaning attached to the symptoms of depression.

The depressive symptoms say that the person as a human being is at a core level. These are much more than just a summary of what the person feels or is struggling within their life at that time.

For many people with eating disorders, depression is strong proof of their unacceptability and guilt, as well as a constant confirmation of the deep level of "flawless" they feel about themselves. The drastic mental reversal of the cognitive distortion of personalization and all-or-nothing mentality magnifies or amplifies the depression's severity. The second sign of major depression shown to be unique in those suffering from severe eating disorders is that their sense of hopelessness and frustration extends far beyond "depressed mood most of the day, sometimes every day." Hopelessness is often an indication of how hollow and incomplete they think about who they are, their life, and their potential. All this hopelessness has been turned into an unhealthy attempt to feel in charge and avoid pain through the excessive acting out of anorexia or bulimia until the eating disorder has been resolved.

Second, this hopelessness can be carried out in recurrent feelings of suicide, omnipresent suicidal ideation, and suicidal behavior that many clients with extreme anorexia and bulimia may have in a more pronounced and ever-present manner than clients with the mood disorder alone. The value of this desire to die and survive is bound up with a much more private sense of self-disdain and denial of personality (get rid of me) than merely wanting to escape the hardships of life. Second, eating disorders are different in the feelings of worthlessness and inadequacy because it reaches beyond those thoughts. It is an identity issue of thoughts of uselessness, futility, and nothingness that arise without the eating disorder's diversion or focus.

A third, unique variable in the depression of those with eating disorders is that their extreme or unnecessary shame is more related to social treatment problems and a feeling of impotence and impotence than can usually be seen in those with major depression. An excruciating self-concern is often in reaction to a failure in their partnerships with significant others to make things unique and good.

The all-consuming essence of anorexia and bulimia is a sixth variable that hides depression in an eating disorder patient. In the course of an eating disorder, there is often a show of high energy coupled with excessive ruminations, compulsiveness, acting out, and the highs and lows. When the eating disorder is eliminated and the patient is no longer in a position or location to carry it out, then the depression is filled in excruciating and obvious ways.

Compassion of Hopelessness

The truth of working with people who struggle with depression or eating disorders is that their hopelessness is hard not to feel helpless. Their lack of hope is particularly excruciating.

It is an internal pain and suffering, supported by deep feelings of self-hatred and self-determination. For many, the eating disorder is supposed to be their mental redemption. It would be thinness, physical beauty, and social acceptance.

Some come to feel they have suffered from the eating disorder or lost their identity in the eating disorder. Therefore, the hopelessness extends beyond hopelessness, because in their life there is not only anything better, there is nothing decent about them. Not only is there no hope for the future, at the present there is nothing optimistic but the frustration we experience is moving in and out.

This seems like the pain is going to last forever. Therapists dealing with eating disorders need to be ready for the depression storm that will come out once the signs or habits of eating disorders have been resolved and reduced to some degree.

It is my observation that therapists need to adjust how they focus on addressing depression in those with eating disorders as relative to those for whom addiction is the main and most important condition. Therapists need to find ways to cultivate optimism for the helpless, much more so for someone with an eating disorder, as they often deny support from these patients.

They want to be happy. We are denying help. They're denying passion. We want to be motivated. We fail to do the stuff that would be most beneficial to bring them out of depression due to their deep inner self-hatred.

The discomfort that fills the room becomes palpable to the psychologist. Clients are often full of sorrow or rage about who they are, contributing to a deeper level of frustration in the symptoms of depression. Working with eating-disordered patients with this depressive degree, the psychologist must display a profound sense of respect, compassion, and love for those who feel so poorly about themselves and who struggle so profoundly in all aspects of their lives.

Such individuals are still willing, amid all the pain, to reach out to others with love and kindness and act at high academic and job performance levels.

They can still be great bosses, workers, or teachers, but in themselves or their life, they cannot find much happiness. Such patients continue to seek secret suffering in life, and the empathy and admiration of a psychologist for this level of determination and perseverance offers a framework of optimism. As counselors, a feeling of love and compassion is vital to develop and is apparent in these moments when the patient experiences nothing but lost or trapped.

Separating Depression from Self-hatred

One of the key components of coping with an eating disorder and depression factors is to start separating the distress from self-hatred. Helping customers understand the difference between guilt and self-hatred is critical. Shame is the false sense of self that drives someone to think or feel that they are inferior, imperfect, deficient, and evil, an internal feeling that something is wrong about their "being."

They feel that they are worthless to the world and themselves and that they somehow lack anything they need to "be enough." Identity-hatred is behaving out of that shame within and outside the individual. Self-hatred can be done in the eating disorder's negative mind, the constant cycle of self-criticism, self-contempt, and dissatisfaction that is a common factor in all eating disorders sufferers.

The guilt can be achieved by self-punishment, self-abandonment, psychological isolation, evasion, minimization, self-harm, self-mutilation, or impulsive and destructive habits both inside and outside the eating disorder.

Self-hatred is the continuing accumulation of information that is distorted or intolerable within the client's head. Over time, the eating disorder is their only confirmation that they are right and that they are undesirable. And so, in a way, their comrade and foe is the eating disorder. It's a source of comfort, and that's why they won't be comforted because until they can achieve perfection in an eating disorder's mindset, they have a great cause to blame themselves for who they are and who they aren't.

All these instances of self-hatred are associated with the signs and speech of depression, so having the person distinguish what depression is and what self-hatred is for them is essential in counseling. My perception has been that concentrating on guilt and self-hatred issues has been more beneficial to those with eating disorders than focusing solely on the depression itself.

Self-hatred amplifies the frequency and performance of depressive symptoms. Through working on the dimensions of self-hatred, they start to turn the volume down on how the depressive symptoms manifest with the patient.

I find that explaining the distinction of self-hatred from depression and its signs and then starting to change and relax the manifestations of self-hatred fosters optimism and brings hope.

Customers start to see and believe that perhaps the problem is not entirely who they are. The optimism comes from knowing that they may not have accurate and true thoughts or a sense of self. We can understand that some of what we have done forever and what a portion of our personality has endured is a self-hatred habit that has been selected and carried out. We start to feel faith for ourselves somewhere in this isolation from self-hatred and despair, hope to let go of suffering, and hope to make our lives sound, appear, and be better.

Another explanation for stressing self-hatred is to help clients start to understand and criticize the unique quality of all-around thinking that leads them in this most destructive, private, and self-contemptuous direction to process everything about their lives.

Hope is created by realizing that everything is not suggesting anything terrible about who they are, that normal life events are not proof of something wrong with them, and that negative feelings are not confirming what they have always believed about themselves as real. The peculiar perfectionism found in this all-or-nothing mentality in any field of thought, emotion, or action leaves little space for anything but ideal. Being willing to let go of the self-hatred barrier to start to see many of these emotions, feelings, and actions that we encounter every day as normal, natural, and reasonable helps to promote hope, particularly the kind of hope that is not bound up with the false hopes of the eating disorder itself. Part of what made the eating disorder stronger is that people poured all their dreams into the eating disorder itself.

Eating disorders were futile because after customers did all they could to fulfill them beautifully, they only added suffering, depression, instability, and more hopelessness. The effort by anorexia and bulimia to create optimism has succeeded.

We continue distinguishing their eating disorder from themselves by dwelling on self-hatred. We continue removing the eating disorder from their source of hope as well. We start recognizing that optimism is within themselves and that hope is within reach when we relax the way they view themselves and change the way they perceive themselves internally and externally.

Separating addiction from self-hatred will help clients see the eating disorder for what it is, with all its myths and implications, and make them start to see who they are more honestly and accurately.

Renaming Depression

I have found it helpful to label and re-frame the depression and its manifestations in some form of common discomfort that they are feeling while dealing with this clientele. They highlight the suffering factors because the internalization of hopelessness is part of what makes depression more unbearable for those with eating disorders. We could strip the international, vague, and potential meaning of depression and divide it into smaller pieces, more concrete, more real, and more psychologically related to their perceptions than to their personality. We're talking a lot about their feelings of pain and grief, or discussing and expanding their perception of being unloved, or their sense of inadequacy, or their feelings of rejection and resentment, etc. In very basic and emotionally connected understandings and words, I seek to explain depression. I rarely speak to them directly regarding their depression while they try to understand, affirm, and create optimism in specific areas of their suffering.

I find it more beneficial to spend sessions about how to build self-esteem over a sense of loss, a sense of powerlessness, a sense of frustration, etc., rather than thinking about depression and what to do to help lessen it.

The reality is that we are both de-amplifying and de-escalating the depression in the course of promoting optimism by reflecting on and addressing the various types of pain. It's difficult to get to the root of the addiction and stop the actual discomfort because ignoring the suffering is what people wanted to do through the eating disorder.

It is important to note here that biochemistry can and is usually involved in the nature, frequency, and form of depression we undergo, and that proper assessment and use of antidepressant drugs is strongly encouraged as an integral part of the treatment.

It is also important to remember that patients with serious eating disorders also avoid substance use or manipulation as an attempt to control their bodies and weight and foster a sense of command.

It is necessary to be very vigilant to periodically track medicine and help to assist patients in the correct understanding of drug usage.

Too often, medication reflects vulnerability and becomes a reason to indulge in self-hatred again rather than being seen as yet another piece of the puzzle that will continue to create confidence for their rehabilitation. It is my understanding that if we can reframe the drug as a positive aspect of their healing and recovery from both depression and an eating disorder, clients frequently react to and benefit from medication.

It is also important to continue evaluating and understanding the effect of poverty on the capacity of clients to perceive and/or change the way they process information about themselves and their life while coping with eating disorders.

Stabilizing the eating disorder as a key treatment and promoting renourishment is necessary before there is any progress in treating depression. Brain and body renourishment is an important early process to promote optimism.

Reducing Loneliness

Getting them out of loneliness is another important component in the treatment of depression by eating disorder clients. Sometimes, re-engaging or reconnecting with other individuals is a very effective technique for customers. Moving away from loneliness and reconnecting in their life with others brings hope.

Pursuing a reconnection with others stresses being responsive to feeling connected, feeling the love, empathy, and concern of others for them, and showing their compassion and love for family members, colleagues, other clients, and clinicians, etc. Involving parents in family therapy, pair relationship buddies, and recovery mates are often very effective ways of reducing depression and raising patient confidence as they feel comforted and encouraged by those who love and care about them. Helping individuals throughout their life to communicate with people again brings hope and the ability to feel something distinct from self-hatred.

Receiving signs of affection, interest, and genuine care for someone else is optimistic and becomes a very important part of depression counseling.

Letting go of False Remorse

Another component of depression treatment has to do with the extreme and irrational degree of remorse. Also, it is because of self-hatred that shame is different for those with eating disorders. The shame encourages them to feel bad or awful for themselves because they are not good, or are not in complete control, or have not been completed, or have not been welcomed and loved by all, or because there are unhappy people in their life.

A suffering that is not going to heal is the misplaced guilt associated with distorted and misleading truths. It's effective in thinking

The fake shame or bad feeling towards themselves is often directly linked to how important people are doing and functioning in their lives. We tend to feel more guilty and accountable for the bad decisions and actions of someone else. False remorse gives them a sense of hopelessness as their desire to alter it or re-frame it is impeded by their self-contempt lens all-around.

They could equate themselves with unrealistic self-standards that no one could live up to, and thus become the exception to all normalcy laws. We have to live beyond reasonable somewhere, and the sense of guilt is proof that they don't operate at the higher level of performance that is anticipated.

Often when they receive suggestions from other people regarding their actions, particularly their eating disorder, experiencing false shame becomes another motivation. The concern with self-inculpation is that it creates intense feelings of remorse, resentment, anger, embarrassment, depression, and sorrow, but it pushes them to self-hatred, self-criticism, self-doubting, and self-punishment instead of pushing them to repentance and improvement.

False shame often contributes to a stronger lack of hope. Releasing false remorse fosters optimism because establishing strong moral limits contributes to an improved sense of freedom and decisions.

Besides, it is important to emphasize that to deal with those with an eating disorder in the field of depression, the frequency and behavior of the eating disorder must first be controlled or reduced. Until we do so, we probably won't see the scope and severity of depression and the very personal nature of how stress presents itself in eating clients with illness.

It is also important to improve our awareness and understanding of how depression is different from those suffering from eating disorders as it offers us treatment choices and a context to engage with those with such coexisting conditions in a more caring and positive manner. The most useful thing we can do with these customers in every session is to build optimism.

Nurturing optimism is not always a simple and straightforward set of strategies and methods, but a desire on the part of both patient and psychologist to confront the hopelessness in a kind and loving environment. I believe such psychological definitions and ideas help to promote more optimism for clients with a coexisting depression or eating disorder. By facing hopelessness, suffering, self-hatred, shame, and loneliness, we will slowly cultivate and create optimism and decrease depression.

New hope contributes to answers. Genuine optimism would lead to a better future. Real optimism is going to bring in improvement.

Depression in youth and kids

I discovered quite a bit of information about depression in particular while doing work on adult depression, in contrast to what I already understood as I struggle with this disorder.

Nonetheless, what I didn't know is just how common this disorder is in the general population, and especially to children and adolescents. One source said depression is close to the western world's top psychological condition (more about what that means in a later blog; it's going to take a whole blog to talk about what that means).

This will address the following: data on teenagers and children with depression; teens and children-specific symptoms of depression (for "normal" symptoms, check out the adult blog), and what you, as a mother and/or guardian, can do if you notice one of the symptoms. Teenager and children depression statistics as many as 8.3 percent of teenagers in the United States are suffering from depression. Suicide is the third leading cause of death by teenagers.

Depression can happen as many as one in every 33 children and about one in eight teenagers. (Mental Health Services Network, 1996; over the last nine years, such numbers have increased).

Major depression medication for adolescents is as successful as it is for adults. (Dr. Graham Emslie, Journal of General Psychiatry, American Medical Association, 15 November 1997).

Depression of adolescents was almost uncommon twenty years ago. Now among young people, there is the highest rate of increase in depression. (I don't know about you, but I am very terrified by this statistic!) The adolescent suicide numbers are sobering. Studies show that one in five (1 in 5) kids has some kind of psychological, cognitive, and emotional disorder, and one in ten (1 in 10) may have a serious emotional issue.

What is even more disturbing is that only 30 percent of all these children and adolescents who deal with emotional and behavioral disorders undergo any kind of therapy and care. The other 70 million only suffer through the stress of mental illness and emotional turmoil, trying their best to reach maturity. Some theorize that this is why teenagers have such a high suicide rate. Suicide is the third (3rd) leading cause of death among 15-24-year-old males. It is the sixth (6th) leading cause of death for children aged 5-14, even more concerning.

The consequences of untreated depression may be increased incidence of adult depression; involvement in the criminal justice system; or suicide in some cases.

What Are the Symptoms of Depression Teen / Children?

Treatment for depression (i.e. counseling, rehabilitation, or even medical intervention if needed) is as successful for adolescents/children as it is for adults, as we see above.

Let me repeat that; evidence from a variety of sources indicates that appropriate treatment for depression is as successful as it is for adults in an adolescent and/or a baby. So, what are we supposed to look for as a parent or guardian? What are the real depression symptoms, not just a "bad mood?"

"True Depression" - the form that needs immediate and proper care— is described in youth and children as when the symptoms of depression linger and interfere with the capacity of the teen/child to cope with their normal daily activities.

This does not mean that if it continues for a couple of days or months, one should disregard the bad mood of a teen/child. What it means is that at least you, the parent/guardian, need to learn enough about the normal daily activities of your teen/child so that you can understand if improvements are taking place.

Okay, what does a teen/child's "normal daily habits" cover? (And here we stick with American standard teens/children because that's what I'm more comfortable with. If anyone can contribute to this book, please do so.) When you go through this document, note that your teen/child must have an "important" amount of these symptoms; they must be persistent, out of character; and hinder the normal daily activities of the teen/child (sound familiar?)

1. Everybody is violently and verbally aggressive.
2. Abandoning everyday activities, beloved interests, and athletics or any other schedule.
3. Improved passive TV viewing (where the teen/child has "thousand-yard exposure" and does not engage with the programs).
4. Increased risk-taking; for example, reckless driving; climbing too high in a tree and falling, destroying something; other particularly risky behaviors.
5. Drug and alcohol misuse. Particularly teenagers who use alcohol and drugs to "escape."
6. Improvements in youth college habits (including training courses and job settings); improvements in pre-school social attitudes and practices (i.e. used to enjoy drawing and playing with clay; now just sitting in the corner, carrying a stuffed toy, and sucking the thumb).
7. Frequent school absences; lower results than historically achieved; decreased skipped classes; etc. For a child, task reversal (i.e., used to draw within the lines, now just scribbling on paper; deliberately breaking items, etc.)
8. Complains to be frustrated (teen); a kid whose concentration waives when not around. A baby who has been seated and concentrating during a community reading suddenly gets up and walks about.
9. Become disruptive in class (both teens and kids).
10. Finds it more difficult to remain on the work. Easily loses concentration; gets distracted psychologically. Finds it hard to make choices. This may appear like the following in a baby: unable to align blocks by color if he/she has been able to play ball before; unable to choose between playing ball

or jumping rope when the child chooses to play ball before. I'm sure you can think about your scenarios.

11. Can't remember promises-don't hold (teen) meetings. As a baby, forget to bring home papers when he/she used to do so; forget home address/telephone number when he/she has known them for months/years; etc.

12. Has trouble standing still or conversely becomes lethargic (sluggish). This would refer to a teen as well as a baby. You may continuously imagine the teen and baby in your mind; jump, move afoot, or both feet; handle things; etc. OR, again watch the teen or babysitting or lying with that thousand yards. AND, yes, this is your teen and child's unusual behavior.

13. Improvements to relationships and partnerships. The transition is typically reflected in aggression and passivity. Arguing if he/she wasn't speaking to you before; or when he/she used to speak to you using the "nothing" response. (Extract that one symptom again; it must be one of many of the signs the adolescent or baby has.)

14. Stop walking with friends; show no interest in community hikes.

15. Rise or decline in sexual activity (the OLDER TEEN, hopefully).

16. Can start to identify with another group of peers (the "evil impact" community as a teenager; the "rowdy" kids as a child).

17. Loses interest in once fun activities.

18. More parental and family disputes than average.

19. Improvements to patterns of eating and sleeping.

20. Expresses excessive remorse, feelings of insufficiency, lack of value, disappointment. (I can see this in a teenager; I don't understand how it would look like in a baby. If you can, please let us know.)

21. Manifest hopelessness and nothing to look forward to.
22. Speak monotonously and monosyllabically.
23. Has a self-concern; is removed.
24. Easy to weep, to appear depressed, to feel alone or disconnected.
25. Become scared of being good.
26. Fearing to do something right. This could appear as bedwetting after YEARS of not bedwetting in a child; fear of darkness or "things going bumping in the night" after YEARS of no depression, etc.
27. self-injury accidents. Ideas for self-murder. (I have no idea how this would feel for a teenager, and expect not to have such an understanding!)

WHAT A PARENT / GUARDIAN CAN DO

The two most important things that a parent can do for your baby/teen are first, KNOW YOUR TEEN / Teenager 'S ROUTINE, AND NORMAL DAILY ACTIVITIES so that you can detect any changes; and, LISTEN:

- listen while your kids are talking;
- listen to their music;
- spend more time with their children;

Of course, but I'm going to say it anyway, understand the above signs and recognize your teen/child. You, the parent or guardian can do some more stuff here.

- Go daily to their daycare to know their schedule; tell the educators to warn you if they adjust their routine.
- If you are a student, go to ALL teacher meetings and understand the dynamics of the normal school day, and demand to be notified for improvements instantly.
- Consider their peers for both teens and children; see if your home can be a "gathering place;" get to consider your

child's and adolescent friends ' parents and promise to let each other know if you see any behavior changes.

- Keep a diary of any improvements you see in any event so that you can discuss the situation with objective consistency and detail if appropriate.
- When you feel your child/teen has issues that can lead to depression, react with compassion, kindness, and support.
- Let your baby or adolescent know you're there whenever he or she wants you, and do so often and in age-specific ways (as Dr. Phil would say).
- If your adolescent locks you out (depressed teens don't want to be patronized or crowded), keep trying, just softly.
- Do not condemn or evaluate when the baby or teen begins to speak (it is vital that he or she talks and shares feelings). REMEMBER, NEVER CRITICIZE FEELINGS; even if you believe they're "correct," everyone has the right to their feelings. Let them be voiced; obtain professional assistance if it is unacceptable.
- Encourage initiatives and support them.
- Get help from a doctor or mental health professional if the distressed feeling of an adolescent or baby does not change with time (be ready to document habits, remember how long or how often they have happened, and how serious they are-hence the above-mentioned diary).
- Don't sit to anticipate the signs to go home alone. It's better to seek support and be assured that your teen/child is fine than having your teen/child become one of the 70 million who never get care.
- If depression becomes serious, seek professional treatment as soon as possible when teenagers and kids are thinking about harming themselves and suicide.

- Depressed teenage parents may need assistance themselves. Check for communities of parents with adolescent depression background.

Drug abuse causes depression in young adolescents is already notorious for their mood swings, defiant actions, and disconnected attitudes, and it is hard to believe that anything could make things worse. At college and in their home lives, adolescents are dealing with a lot, except for their emotions going' out of whack.' It has been proven that adolescents not only seek more medications in their teenage years than at any other time in their lives (over 70%), but the side effects and long-term effects of this practice are dangerous and sometimes fatal.

Many early indications that your adolescent son or daughter may use drugs may include, but are not restricted to:* Noticeable shifts in dress and/or appearance* Tardiness at work, home, classes, and/or family activities* Secretive behavior, including a majority of time spending alone behind closed doors* Spending time with new friends; many time friends prefer to keep a secret* Grades falling.

Sometimes by consuming and/or abusing drugs or alcohol, a youth can slip into a fitting in hole.

The factor teenagers prefer to use or misuse drugs or alcohol is the same as adults; they try to avoid problems or feelings in real life. High-stress home lives, getting teased at school, losing college scores, etc. all can create an easy escape for an adolescent.

Noticing these causes and supporting your teen with issues, then, can prevent them from abusing a drug to fix the problem temporarily.

Drugs and alcohol in teenagers have since been shown to cause long-lasting depression. It has also been related to suicide rates by teens across the United States since this finding. Suicide rates are currently the third highest cause of death for teens across the U.S.

Such numbers are alarming, but knowing what the suicidal tendencies come from is important.

What researchers found was that the depression is linked to the drug or alcohol itself only in part. The main reason for signs of depression was that teens realized it was contradictory to what their parents expected from them, and therefore, shame leads to depression.

Trying to get to know your teenager better every day is vital. Of course, they won't give you all the knowledge that bounces around in their heads, but a parent-child partnership must build connections and trust.

When the teenager has an unhealthy addiction to drugs and liquor, visiting a drug and alcohol rehabilitation center is always in your interest. There's no fear trying to change the problem early, and it's a wise decision to gain valuable knowledge about your child's welfare.

How Teenage Depression Affects Teenage Self-Esteem

Depression among adolescents is a common problem facing many adolescents. Even if they come from the healthiest setting, various hormonal changes to their body result in them feeling extremely low or discouraged.

When parents do not take it seriously it can result in loss of teenage self-esteem and eventually teens can take extreme measures by committing suicide.

It is therefore important to give teens lots of love and unquestioned support to help them get through this tough period of their life. Here are some of the signs that can help you determine if your child is experiencing depression.

Behavioral Symptoms: Poor adolescent self-esteem and teenage depression may show themselves in the form of extreme behavioral traits including avoidance and irritable behavior or increased violence. We might get angry about the smallest of things and start shouting.

Sometimes they can drop things in the house and destroy them in other ways. In some other situations, they may disappear entirely and stop communicating with family members.

Suicidal Thoughts and Self-Harm: Suicidal tendencies and self-harm are both severe signs of adolescent depression and poor youth self-esteem.

The Following is some of the main signs of suicidal impulses and self-harm:

- Your adolescent begins thinking about contemplating suicide
- They begin associating with death in a meaningful way
- Some teens often go further by fantasizing about death by private diaries or poetry or posting posts on social networking platforms showing their thoughts
- Others demonstrate careless behavior like driving too fast, hurting themselves, and having a lot of accidents
- Your teenager might also start withdrawing from best friends and family
- They can seek weapons and materials to commit suicide
- Self-harm can be noticed by cuts or scarring, a tendency to wear a different style of clothing to cover up the marks, or finding sharp objects or plasters in your teen's room.

Such habits are very dangerous and as parents, you need to take your child to a doctor or therapist instantly.

Eating Disorders: One major symptom of adolescent depression is eating disorders due to severe weight gain or loss. Low adolescent self-esteem stemming from health, overweight and poor performance at college can drive some teens to go to the extreme of either consuming too much or too little. When you start noticing these signs, it is worth checking to see if the child is suffering from depression.

Youth depression is one of the biggest causes of past youth suicides. Families must be extremely careful to offer their teens full help so that they can safely navigate through this tough time of their lives. More than 100 resources were given in the book "Solving Teenage Issues" to help parents accept their adolescents who have depression or any other adolescent issues that lead to depression. Parents must use every resource to keep their teens satisfied beyond their means.

Clinical Signs of Teenage Depression in Teenage Girls

Clinical signs of depression in adolescent girls can be difficult to recognize or interpret based on ordinary behaviors and behavior that most adolescent girls display from day today.

Nevertheless, with teen suicide on the increase in women, parents need to remain alert and never take anything for granted. Depression in teenagers is possible and can be severe.

It's even worse for the teen to deal with as difficult as adolescent depression is to remember. Many teenage girls who experience severe depression and don't get treatment often have a far better chance of falling in with the wrong crowd, struggling at college, becoming involved in drugs, being promiscuous, or trying to commit suicide.

Furthermore, adolescents who experience depression and don't receive help for the rest of their lives can maintain any portion of the disorder. Recognizing the psychiatric signs of depression in adolescent girls and seeking medical assistance for those showing such signs should be the priority of every adolescent girl's family.

Medical symptoms of depression in teenage girls

Clinical signs of depression in teenage girls frequently verge on normal emotions, but if the following signs occur for more than a month, you or your daughter must visit a doctor;

social awkwardness and isolation: when a teenage girl feels unable to mingle with social commitments without feelings of inferiority, she is insecure. Peer pressure becomes extremely difficult for teens and the fear of rejection.

Socially awkward teens tend to avoid social situations. Her loss of interest means that she feels like an outcast or that she believes she is unworthy of love.

Grief, Death, and Thoughts of Suicide: Teen girls seem to find it difficult to cope with death-related grief and problems. A family tragedy may lead a teen girl to fall into despair as easily as a pet's death or a relationship failure or a partner breaks up. If your baby is depressed and withdrawn or has thoughts of suicide, be vigilant, and seek medical assistance.

Low self-esteem: We are often admitted to classes if adolescent girls are anxious, which also tend to be unhealthy at some point or are involved in drugs or promiscuous behavior. When this occurs, she can believe that this sort of party is the only type of love she may get or is deserving to receive.

Depression, frustration, irritability, and despair are typical signs of depression. Documenting the mood swings of your baby may be as time-consuming as it may be monotonous, but if your child does not open up to you, this may be the best way to understand what may occur inside the mind of your child.

If your daughter throws tantrums, is violent, and/or does not seem to be able to control her impulses, the first signs of depression may be looked at.

Poor performance and poor concentration: grades at college will decrease when concentration and focus are scattered.

Disrupted sleep habits, health, and energy loss: once sleep patterns are disturbed, symptoms of tiredness generally follow. It is also possible to hear signs of nausea, stomachs, and other physical ailments.

Loss in appetite: there may be no feeding or binge eating.

Remorse: There may also be intense feelings of guilt and hopelessness suggesting that your child needs help.

Because each baby is unique and because there are always external influences and precursors to this disorder, such as genes and peer pressure, nothing is taken for granted.

Since biology plays a part in this process, the baby may be genetically wired for some of the same illnesses if you or your partner or someone else in the community have undergone a form of depression.

So, if your child shows any of these symptoms or participates in abnormal activities for her, seek advice from the doctor of your family.

Coping with Depression

If you consider a form of depression in your baby, the first and most important thing to do is seek medical attention. A trained professional will be able to tell you what symptoms to watch for and when such signs indicate an illness.

Pay attention to her mood swings and benefit from her emotional outbursts and periods of solitude and know which things are too much for your mother to bear. A child who unexpectedly is withdrawn and finds safe harbor in her space may experience daunting challenges that may need your advice. And whenever a teenage girl is fascinated with death and experimentation on her own body with any sort of mutilation such as cutting or burning herself, it's time for you to get professional help.

Ways to Prevent Depression in Teen Girls

Parents are in a tough place. The normal individual is not trained to recognize the signs of depression in adolescent girls, and sometimes the signs are so minute that even parents who are attentive to the temperament of their daughter do not see problems for what they are.

Understanding your mother as well as you can is the best way to understand that something is going on with your child. Keep the family together by working together as a group in sports, but also set aside time for you and your wife.

Moms who spend time with their daughter shopping and doing other hobbies together often have a strong connection.

Daughters can and should also be communicating with their mothers. As a young girl's father, you can connect with her and her mom in the same way, or you can find other ways to spend time together. Take responsibility, for instance, to teach your daughter to ride. In the meantime, show her a car's mechanics how to patch a tire, change the oil, or pump gas, and spend time with her telling her about one of your private hobbies.

Share with her, and she will share with you most of the time in exchange. As issues escalate, a teenage girl who has someone to open up with when she has an issue will have a defense mechanism already in motion.

Any adolescent girl who does not have that mechanism in place will have a tougher time dealing with problems and may potentially become seriously depressed.

Helping Teenagers

Growing up as a teenager is one of the most frustrating and challenging times in an individual's life. Tragically assumed depression in teenagers in this day and age is all too normal.

In the form of depression, a mixture of raging hormones, body image, peer pressure, family tension, and pressure to perform well at college may take their toll on adolescents. Read on to read some tips to help adolescents deal with their depression and rebound from it.

Drastic Strategies to Assist Teenagers with Depression

1) *Psychological Assistance*-There's so much going on in your life as an adolescent right now that it can get very complicated and stressful. A must is that you have some kind of social support during this tough time, whether you're speaking to your family, friends, peers, or even a supportive educator or school counselor. Make sure that there is someone you can offer your thoughts and feelings to as this practice alone will take away massive pressure from you and is a basic form of therapy. You will always seem so much larger in your mind, whatever may be disturbing, but once you write it out to someone else it usually loses the bite.

2) *Do what you like* make sure you get a chance to do something you like doing as often as possible. A game and recreation you love can help keep your depression away while you relieve your stress and tension and can be your true self. This can be very relaxing and I want you to find time for this every day.

3) *Don't deal with being sad*-this is a big problem most depressed people face, but they don't realize they're doing it. Depression must be seen as a transitional phase you're passing through and not as something you're dealing with.

54

It becomes part of you when you connect with it, and then it will always be there irrespective of what you do, the same way you identify with both an arm and a leg.

A way to break out of this self-identification of depression is to say that you are not a survivor, because psychologically it removes the depression from your self-image of yourself and renders it a different entity from which you can now isolate yourself.

Do that now! "I'm not a survivor," I think you've been motivated by this guidance on depression in youth. Feel free to read it all over again and make sure you understand everything as I hope that this information can benefit you, even a little bit.

Teenage Depression Cured by Hypnosis

Teenage Depression is not just unpleasant moods or depression from time to time. Depression is a serious issue affecting any part of a teen's existence. In class, family, and life in general, it can lead to problems. As recently noted in the media, teens who committed suicide believed to be induced by cyberbullying can even contribute to disaster.

Cyberbullying is fresh and can extend to hundreds of children quickly. It's like ripples in the water and there's no clear way of controlling it. If you are the target of this kind of harassment, you may start to feel like the whole universe is against you and have no room to turn around.

When you feel your teen spends too much time on the internet and seems to be excessively moody, you may be searching for some of these signs of depression: frustration & restlessness Feelings of worthlessness or remorse Feelings of lack of enthusiasm and determination Irritability, rage, or aggression Hopelessness and disappointment Loss of interest in activities Teen depression looks different than adult depression and it can kill their growing identity because they still figure out who they are. If they are the victim of bullying, whether on the internet or in life, it can contribute to an intense sense of sadness, frustration, and rage, and sometimes even suicide, as has been the case recently in the media.

Experts say that 1 in 5 teenagers who are troubled receive assistance. Teenagers may be afraid to tell their family they're sad or have school issues, but sadly they're dependent on their parents and educators so they can't seek help on their own so they don't ask for it most of the time. We fear we might be letting down their family or not respecting them.

If you have a teenager in your life, knowing what youth depression looks like and what to do if you notice the warning signs is crucial.

We might withdraw from relationships and events, or they may start hanging with another group.

They might have moods that are irritable and frustrated, grumpy and aggressive, and susceptible to angry outbursts.

You may have debilitating nausea, vomiting, and stomach pains.

We may have an intense technical vulnerability and may feel worthless or ignored.

They can run away, self-medicate with drugs and alcohol, become abusive, or have reckless behavior to deal with their emotional pain. Or they might go the other way and try to avoid using or isolating unnecessary machines. Depression may cause school grades to fall, poor attendance, and low self-esteem. We may even experience eating disorders and conditions of self-injury at times.

Speak with them if you believe that your teen is going through some difficult times. Don't be afraid to voice your worry. Even if they don't answer right away, they need to feel you care. You can get help from a therapist you know and think that can help you get your teen back on track. Make sure that your adolescent is involved in sports or other sporting events, perhaps even charity service or mentoring programs.

Depressed or Lazy?

Anyone with a youth understands they are inspired by the constant battle. The constant struggle with adolescent years ' laziness and non-cooperation. They should remain vigilant as parents to be certain they are sad and lazy.

The rate of depression for teenagers is very high. With all the additional hormonal tension, social pressure, tasks, and assignments along with any extra school events, it's no wonder. Remove the fear of failure and the desire to know what to do with the rest of your life.

The symptoms of depression in teens are different from depression in adults or children. Often these signals make them appear as if they were slow.

They may not even know, sadly, that they are sad. Children won't have the concept of needing help if they don't know how bad a condition it is. It's most likely up to the adults in their lives to find out if they're genuinely sad and lazy. To do this, the signs of depression in youth must be identified and remembered.

Such indicators can differ from one gender to another, but there are some indications similar to both male and female teenagers.

Signs of depression are typically normal to both sexes:

- excessively negative antisocial actions
- Retreating frequently to their rooms and wanting to leave their presence with carelessness at work.
- Disinterest in experiences or events with the parents.

Depression symptoms are typically more common in men: excessive hostility and anger.

- Reckless behavior involving the abuse of illegal substances

Symptoms of depression are typically more prevalent in females:

- Being messy in a presentation.
- A new or unusual fear about mortality or suicide.
- Negative activity with the opposite sex (whether promiscuous or separated from them)

Some Other Symptoms That Might Appear:

- lower self-esteem than usual suicidal comparisons (in some extreme cases)
- A general negative life view.

While teenagers strive to be autonomous, they will need support from a youth dealing with depression. It's probably up to you to force them to unlock their feelings. At least enough to be able to decide what kind of assistance to give.

Stay upfront with any suggestions to explore and deal with depression in your child. Inform them that their recent behavior bothers you. Think with depression, make sure it's a treatable disease.

When their depression is serious, and they think about suicide, wanting to die, etc.

Talk to your friends and family if your teen won't talk to you. For their issues, they may have opened up to them.

Recommend by giving a favorite activity or trip for one-on-one space. Tell them specifically if they need to think about anything.

Don't bring them on an illusion, just let them know about you.

Stay cautious. Look for signs of depression and if you see them, take extreme action. Take the time to be there for them and listen when they call out.

The only way to be sure is to be observant if the adolescent is sad and lazy. Watch carefully for behavioral changes. Despite usually being good at hiding depression from us, this should help you catch it early.

Depression and gender

Two-thirds of all individuals suffering from depression are females for purposes that are not well known. For this reality, researchers suggested biological, psychological, and cultural reasons.

The biological theory is based on the fact that females appear to be at higher danger of depression when their hormone concentrations alter considerably, as they did during the premenstrual era, the period after a child's birth, and menopause start. Throughout their lives, the hormone concentrations of men tend to stay more stable.

Therefore, researchers theorized that females are naturally at a higher danger of depression. Yet the proof is either incompatible or opposite to support this hypothesis.

Although adolescent and adult women have been discovered to encounter depression twice as high as men, the college population appears to be a significant exception, with men and women experiencing equivalent levels. Why? For this anomaly, several theories have been proposed.

The university campus ' cultural organizations provide males and females with a more egalitarian gender role status.

Women in college have fewer adverse occurrences than females in high college. College males report more adverse occurrences than high school males.

College females report lower social networks that are more sympathetic. A stressful occurrence often precedes depression. Therefore, some psychologists theorized that females could be more stressed than males and therefore more likely to become depressed.

Women, however, do not report more stressful occurrences than males do. Finally, scientists noted variations in gender in coping strategies or the reaction to certain occurrences or stimuli and suggested the argument that women's approaches placed them at a greater danger of depression than men's approaches.

College students were questioned to show how probable they were to participate in the conduct described in each item on the list, presented with "a list of items individuals do when depressed."

Men were more inclined to argue that, "I stop talking about why I'm depressed," "I'm doing something physical," or "I'm playing sports." Women were more inclined to argue that, "I'm trying to determine why I'm depressed," "I'm talking about my emotions to other individuals," and "I'm crying to alleviate stress."

If concentrating on depressed emotions intensifies these emotions, they may be more probable to become clinically depressed by the reaction type of women than males.

There has been no direct testing of this theory, but some supporting proof indicates its legitimacy.

Why are women twice as depressed as men?

It struck me in my face like a pot of ice-water. I put a book back this morning and it came open to this: the levels of depression for contemporary Western females are half that for males.

How might that be? We have access to previous generations ' unprecedented autonomy, careers, schooling, birth control, treatment, and choices. What's going to get us? What is so much bugging us? I finished cleaning up and started reading.

Can these be our hormones? Nope. While hormonal variables may play a part in feeling lousy, the whopping distinction between males and females is not important enough to account for.

Genetics? Maybe for some old developmental purpose, we're just predisposed? That also doesn't justify it. While there is a tendency for generations to pass on depression, careful genetic examination shows that such a wildly lopsided disproportion cannot be accounted for.

How about our desire to speak more publicly than males about our depression? No, even when individuals who are very private about their inner countries are being researched, the two-to-one proportion appears.

Maybe it's because females go beyond males to treatment, so it's more publicized and researched? While we do, the same outcome comes from door-to-door studies. Women who are not in treatment have half the levels of depression as males who are not in treatment.

Is it because of discrimination based on sex, or because of financial variables, since females tend to have worse employment for less cash? No. Women are twice as depressed as males, rich or poor, well-employed or unemployed.

How about the various requirements and functions females face today, plus managing kids and keeping a house? Nor does this hypothesis pan out. Working women are less depressed than residents, with fewer requirements imposed on them.

One by one, in "What You Can Change & What You Can't, A Guide to Successful Self-Improvement," Martin Seligman eliminates the potential culprits. Seligman is regarded as the "dad of constructive parenting" and has written and studied widely on pleasure and how to attain it. He provides three feasible reasons after hunting down all the apparent opportunities, all of which are verified by social science.

The proof points to this: First, taught helplessness, a demonstrated predictor of depression, is much more common in females than in males. We often feel that we have no power over a situation's result, even if we can regulate it because we have "discovered" that we are helpless.

Seligman suggests females receive a masterful education in helplessness-boys learning to be active and creative, girls learning to be passive and dependent, from cradle to grave. Our culture devalues females who become husbands and mothers, and females who do not marry or have kids are viewed as out of location.

Sisters, how about this one? Women who are successful or powerful are seen as hard, bitchy, and aggressive. Man-like. Who likes it? Not me, not me. So why worry, we're telling ourselves and ignoring our soul's yearnings.

Because if we are doomed and doomed if we are not, we tend to give up and stop attempting. We suppose that when we are helpless, we are not helpless.

Second, we're ruminating more, churning and worrying about our upsets and their triggers, much more than people are doing.

We are losing our employment and want to understand why, what we have done wrong, what has occurred, how we could have avoided it, who has not liked us, and on and on. This type of reflection is unnecessary and digs us into a profound mental hole.

Men tend to disregard and take intervention, causation, and exploration. It may not be good action— they may get drunk, watch sports, or distract themselves otherwise. But inside they don't churn about it.

Sound like this in our internal worlds: will he call? He may not like me. What was incorrect with me? That was the incorrect thing I said. I wish she hadn't been angry. How can I remedy it? I haven't done enough. I've been doing too much. I'm not sufficient.

Sounds like this in the inner world of a man: Hmmm, wonder what's in the fridge? TGIF. Tonight, can't wait for the match. Maybe I'm going to call that woman with whom I came out.

Do I guess I'm kidding? Ask a guy. I have. Lots of moments. And they are telling me these types of responses regularly. Sure, they're also worried. They're ruminating, of course. But we don't like that.

Third, the useless pursuit of thinness (and this one was the large shocker for me, so shut up, ladies). Yep. With such zeal that we have depressed ourselves in record amounts, we are pursuing a biologically impossible dream. We hate so much of our natural curves. We strive to have such an unnaturally slim body that we work up into astonishing and unprecedented quantities of depression excessively, fruitlessly, and unhealthily.

Hormones give them lean bodies when kids reach puberty; when women come, we get body fat. What do you think? We need that additional fat to build estrogen and female hormones that bless us with smooth, soft hair, soft bodies, children, and breast milk as well.

How are we going to answer this donation? We hatred, hunger, vomit, workout, concern, lipo, pummel and then overflow into a huge depression.

In believing that our natural beauty is hideous, we are brainwashed by ourselves and our society.

Here's a strong factoid: every culture on the planet that thinks slender females to be perfect has females more likely to experience depression and an eating disorder. Any world culture not worshiping the unnaturally slender female body at the altar has no eating disorders and no lopsided female-to-male depression.

Please be evident on this one. I don't suggest that eating too much is an emotionally sound choice. But it's futile and extremely self-destructive to torture ourselves because we don't have a body like a prepubescent teenager, loathing our lovely, curvy, obviously gentle bodies. And our addiction adds to a climate that transmits this point of view to our kids, who start "dieting" almost as quickly as they learn to read and write.

What's the nice news about it all?

It can change all three of these triggers. Learned impotence, rumination, and poor body image are all based on habits of thinking and fake convictions we can regulate and alter. All of them by themselves.

Isn't this incredible, fantastic, fantastic news? I'm going to tell you that again. Modern Western women's significant causes of depression can be altered by altering our thinking. We have power over things by altering something.

I don't know about you, but it was the most powerful finding I've ever build to learn that I controlled most of the stuff that bugged and annoyed me. And I'm not lightly saying that. I'm a lawyer. I earned instances when I practiced law that had an impact on the life of thousands of people. I'm a mom. I gave birth to two drug-free kids at home and linked with the torrential forces of my body.

These two roles brought me tremendous energy and happy emotions.

But the strength and happiness accessible through handling my self-destructive habits of thinking was beyond anything I've ever encountered, and beyond anything, I've ever thought.

Once I got the hang of it - with easy instruments that are strong, user-friendly, and available-my lifelong urges to feel powerless, care excessively, and hate myself for not being constructed like a Barbie doll started to fade away. It hasn't come back so far.

So, ladies, what are you saying? Are we going to declare a ceasefire on us and our bodies? Is it acceptable for some of us to have breasts and hips, and, ahem, muffin tops, and that's all right?

OCD Depression

OCD sufferers have been discovered to benefit from depression in many distinct instances apart from OCD. While there is still to be defined as the accurate scientific connection between OCD and depression, most specialists agree that individuals with OCD also have a greater likelihood of creating other mental illnesses.

OCD's most prevalent partner was Major Depressive Disorder. The alarming reality behind this is the most probable failure of his OCD therapy when a patient is depressed.

The diagnosis provided to an individual who abruptly stops to appreciate the operations he or she used to love doing is a major depressive disorder. This is more than just feeling sad or blue as the disease can go directly for at least two weeks to a horrible extent like pulling the individual into serious sadness or weariness every day!

The individual will most probably consume little or worse for at least two weeks, refuse to consume as a result of illness or serious weight loss. In other cases, the person will indulge in eating too much in a short time to the point of gaining a lot of weight.

An individual with a major depressive disorder will either sleep much or sleepless, think unless they are fragile, slow, fidgety, or guilty. And a sufferer will have recurring ideas of suicide and mortality in most instances!

Statistically speaking, two out of every three OCD patients will encounter at least one episode of major depression throughout their entire lives. The depression happens in most instances after the ritual achievement is produced or curbed. The likely explanation for this is the ongoing distress caused by self-pressure and its environment vis-à-vis its ritual of OCD.

However, specialists proceed to claim that the close link between major depressive disorder and OCD may be due to two variables: (1) biological and (2) psychological. This result is reached after it has been discovered that the same areas in the brain display pattern modifications for both illnesses. Now, depression is widely regarded as the reaction of the brain to the annoying need to do some obsessions and compulsions.

To better assist his rehabilitation from his OCD, it is very essential to identify the causes of the depressive conduct of an OCD sufferer. Severe depression is probable to interfere with today's OCD medicines. If an OCD physician is well conscious of the patient's situation, i.e. his depressive conduct, then he or she can tailor a program or treatment specifically intended to satisfy the requirements of the patient's situation.

In addition to hypnosis, therapies such as exposure and response prevention are among the most prevalent therapists significantly impaired by depression ineffectiveness. However, it is discovered that depression does not affect the efficacy of medicines and drugs such as SSRIs. This type of therapy is used in instances where depression is present.

Old age and depression Most males and females aged 55-74 report being happy with their life and in excellent health at the moment. While the elderly may experience periods of depression, it is essential to note that this is not an ordinary component of aging.

Depression is the most prevalent mental health problem among elderly adolescents, influencing 15 to 20 percent of the community's elderly people.

It's not a standard aging component. Symptoms such as reduced energy, bad sleep, and health concerns should be considered as feasible diseases of a treatable disease and are NOT the consequence of the aging process.

Depression treatment operates, yet too many individuals stay undiagnosed and untreated because the signs and symptoms of depression are not recognized.

The following definition of major depression is usually agreed upon by mental health experts: symptoms continue for two weeks or longer People either have depressed moods or appear unable to appreciate life.

Major depression should be regarded if four of the following seven requirements are present: a shift in sleeping patterns (more or less than normal) A shift in eating practices or weigh low-energy or fatigue concentration disorder Feeling useless or excessively guilty Marked restlessness or slow-down motions Death thoughts or suicide Depression can be described as a brain chemicals imbalance.

Depression is NOT a personality or character defect.

Many of the signs of depression may also suggest other issues or medical circumstances-it is essential to consult a doctor to determine if depression or other medical condition indicates your diseases.

Depression is often hard to acknowledge among the elderly and continues to be diagnosed. Not only does living with depression prevent older adults from fully enjoying their life, but it also brings a burden on their health, which may contribute to other medical issues. It's also very hard for their caregivers and also puts a burden on their health.

What we do understand is that there is no single source for depression— every person is distinctive in what can cause depression and what can trigger a depressive event. Genetics and family history, brain chemistry, character, significant disease, drugs & alcohol, and life activities are some feasible causes and risk variables. Risk considerations for severe depression can include loss and bereavement, absence of social support, isolation, residing in poverty, being a caregiver, and violence, especially in older adults.

Depression, especially in elderly men, may also boost the danger of suicide among older adults. Seniors account for over 16 percent of all suicide fatalities, according to the CDC. Older adults over the era of 60 are much more probable than older individuals to have a greater likelihood of suicide. If you think a friend or loved one is suicidal, promote them to seek assistance from either a doctor, a friend, a crisis center, or an organization for mental health.

Keep in mind some stuff: maintain a favorable approach. Remember, slowing down doesn't imply you're going to have to stop completely. Chances are you're still going to be able to do almost all the stuff you used to do; you might just need to spend a little more time and discover how to keep track.

See your doctor from your family frequently. Then he/she can handle any modifications or diseases that involve medical care.

Be cautious with your medicines. As you get older, they may start to communicate with other medicines differently and have different effects on you than before. Make sure that your physician understands all of your medicines, including those recommended by another physician.

Responsible for your safety. Do not hesitate to request questions from your physician; unless questioned, some will not give reasons.

Depression is a severe treatable disease. Furthermore, it can be overwhelming for a caregiver to deal with a person who is suffering from depression or in danger of suicide. Although the caregiver provides their loved ones with support and support, they also need to look after their own emotional, mental, and physical well-being.

Although from moment to moment we may all think sad, sorrow is not depression, and it is essential to note that depression is not an ordinary component of aging.

Approximately 80% of all serious instances concerning anorexia or bulimia have a coexisting significant diagnosis of depression. Depression is in and of itself a very painful and all-consuming disease. Depression, however, is beyond devastation in conjunction with an eating disorder and is often disguised within the eating disorder itself. Depression appears different in eating disorder clients than it does in mood disturbance clients alone.

One way to define how depression appears in an eating disorder sufferer is concealed poverty.

For eating disorder clients, depression takes on a heightened quality of hopelessness and self-hatred and becomes an expression of their identity, not a list of unpleasant symptoms.

Depression becomes intertwined with eating disorder manifestations, and the depressive signs are often not distinguishable from the eating disorder due to this interwoven nature. One aim of this paper is to show some of the similarities and distinctions in how depression is manifested in someone with anorexia or bulimia. Another aim is to provide recommendations that start fostering hope within the treatment environment for these desperate clients.

When coping with instances of eating illness, it is essential to realize that it is most probably present at two stages if major depression is present. First, a history of chronic, low-level, dysthymic depression will be obvious, and second, symptoms will be compatible with one or more extended episodes of acute major depressive disorder. The depression's severity and acuteness are not always identifiable instantly in how the customer manifests their eating disorder. Taking clinical history will show acute discouragement, emotions of inadequacy, poor self-esteem, appetite disruption, sleep disruption, poor energy, fatigue, concentration difficulties, decision-making difficulties, and a particular sense of unhappiness and vague desperation.

Since most eating disorder clients have not been seeking therapy for many years, it is not unusual for this type of acute dysthymic depression to have been from two to eight years in their life anywhere. Clinical history will also show that there is a concomitant history of intense signs of major depression as the eating disorder escalated or became more serious in its severity.

In those with long-standing eating disorders, recurrent episodes of major depression are often seen. Simply put, eating disorder clients have long been discouraged, they have not felt nice about themselves for a lengthy moment, they have long felt desperate, and they have experienced aggressive times of depression in which life has become much worse and harder for them.

Unique features an intense and elevated amount of self-hatred and self-contempt is one of the most special features of depression in someone suffering from an eating disorder. This may be because those with these major depressive episodes in combination with an eating disorder have a much more personal adverse and identity-based significance connected to the signs of depression.

The depressive signs claim that the individual as a human being is at a key stage. They are much more than just a description of what the person experiences or are getting from in their lives at that moment. For many females with eating disorders, depression is wide evidence of their unacceptability and shame, as well as regular evidence of the profound stage of "flawed news" they think in themselves. This severe perceptual twist of the cognitive distortion of personalization and all-or-nothing thinking magnifies or amplifies the depression's strength. The second symptom of major depression shown to be distinct in those suffering from serious eating disorders is that their feeling of hopelessness and desperation extends far beyond "depressed mood most of the day, almost every day."

Hopelessness is often an illustration of how empty and hopeless they feel about who they are, their life, and their future. All this hopelessness has been transformed into an addictive effort to stay in command or prevent pain through the obsessive working out of anorexia or bulimia until the eating disorder has been settled.

Third, this hopelessness can be carried out in recurring ideas of suicide, omnipresent suicidal ideation, and suicidal gesture that many clients with serious anorexia and bulimia may have in a more reinforced and ever-present fashion than clients with the mood disorder alone. The quality of this desire to kill or die is bound up with a much more private feeling of self-disdain and denial of identity (get rid of me) than simply wanting to flee the problems of life. Fourth, eating diseases are special in the emotions of worthlessness or inadequacy because it gets beyond those emotions. It is an identification problem with emotions of uselessness, futility, and nothingness that happen without the eating disorder's diversion and obsession.

A fifth, separate part in the depression of those with an eating disorder is that their unnecessary and inappropriate guilt is more linked to mental care problems and a feeling of impotence or impotence than can typically be seen in those with major depression. Their painful self-concern is often in reaction to their failure in their interactions with important others to build things new or better.

The all-consuming nature of anorexia and bulimia is a sixth variable that masks depression in an eating disorder client. There is often a show of elevated energy in the process of an eating disorder connected with obsessive ruminations, compulsiveness, working out, and the highs and lows. When the eating disease is removed and the person is no longer in a situation or location to carry it out, then the depression is flooded in painful and obvious forms.

For many, the eating disorder was supposed to be their mental salvation. It would be thinness, physical perfection, or personal acceptance. Many come to think they even failed in the learning disorder and missed their place in the eating disorder. Therefore, the hopelessness extends beyond hopelessness, because in their life there is not only anything decent, there is nothing good in them.

Not only is there no hope for the future, at the moment there is nothing hopeful but the desperation they feel is breathing in and out. It looks like the pain is going to last indefinitely. Therapists working with eating disorders need to be prepared for the depression flood that will pour out once the symptoms and patterns of eating disorders have been stabilized or limited to some extent.

It is my private remark that clinicians need to modify what they emphasize when managing depression in those with eating disorders rehabilitation as opposed to those for whom depression is the main and most important disease. Therapists need to discover methods to promote hope for the desperate, much more so for someone with an eating illness, as they often seek convenience from these clients. They hesitate to be comfortable. They are refusing assistance. They're rejecting love. They hesitate to be encouraged. They hesitate to do the stuff that would be most useful to lift them out of depression due to their severe internal self-hatred.

The suffering that enters the space is concrete to the doctor. Clients are often full of sadness and rage about who they are, leading to a greater stage of desperation in the symptoms of depression. Working with eating-disordered clients with this depression stage, the doctor needs to demonstrate a profound feeling of regard, gratitude, and love for those who feel so negatively about themselves and who suffer so greatly in all parts of their life. These individuals are still willing, despite all the pain, to reach out to others with love and compassion and operate at elevated educational and job efficiency concentrations.

They can still be wonderful employers, employees, and students, but in themselves or their lives, they cannot discover any happiness. These clients tend to pursue concealed poverty in their lives, and the empathy and consideration of a therapist for this stage of determination and perseverance offers a context for hope.

As therapists, a feeling of affection and compassion is essential to growing and is obvious in these moments when the client feels nothing but desperate and trapped. Self-hatred can be performed in the eating disorder's adverse mind, that constant circle of self-criticism, self-contempt, and negativity that is a prevalent variable in all eating disorders sufferers. The shame can be accomplished through self-punishment, self-abandonment, mental rejection, prevention, minimization, self-harm, self-mutilation, and impulsive and addictive actions both inside and outside the eating disorder.

Self-hatred is the continuing collection of proof that is violated and inappropriate within the client's mind. In a moment, the eating disease becomes their primary proof that they are incorrect and that they are inappropriate. And so, in a way, their friend and foe is the eating disorder. It's a source of comfort, and that's why they won't be comforted, and until they can achieve perfection in an eating disorder's mindset, they have a great cause to hate themselves for who they are and who they aren't.

All these instances of self-hatred become intertwined with the signs and manifestation of depression, thus helping the client distinguish what depression is and what self-hatred is for them becomes essential in treatment. My knowledge has been that concentrating on shame and self-hatred elements has been more helpful to those with an eating disorder than concentrating solely on the depression itself. Self-hatred amplifies the depressive signs' strength and quality. By concentrating on the elements of self-hatred, we start to turn the volume down on how the depressive signs appear with the customer.

Some hope arises from understanding that they may not have precise and real emotions and feelings of self. They may acknowledge that some of what they have accomplished indefinitely and what a portion of their personality has felt is a self-hatred model that has been selected and carried out.

They start to find faith in themselves somewhere in this division of self-hatred and depression, hope to let go of pain, and hope to make their lives feel, look, and be distinct.

Another reason for emphasizing self-hatred is to assist clients to start to acknowledge and question the distinctive value of all-around thinking that causes them in this most adverse, private, and self-contemptuous manner to filter everything about their life.

Hope is produced by understanding that everything is not saying something poor about who they are, that normal life experiences are not proof of something incorrect with them, and that adverse emotions are not proving what they have always felt about themselves as real. The distinctive perfectionism intrinsic in this all-

or-nothing concept in any region of thought, sensation, or conduct enables no space for anything but perfection.

Being willing to let go of the self-hatred filter and start to see many of these ideas, emotions, and actions that they encounter every day as typical, normal, and acceptable starts to promote trust, especially the kind of hope that is not bound up with the fake hopes of the eating disorder itself. Part of what made the eating disorder so strong is that clients placed all their hopes into the eating disorder itself. Eating disorders are hopeless because after clients have done everything in their power to live them perfectly, they have only brought misery, despair, dysfunction, and more hopelessness. The effort by anorexia and bulimia to build hope has failed. They start to distinguish their eating disorder from themselves by concentrating on self-hatred. They start separating the eating disease from their source of hope as well.

They start recognizing that trust is within themselves and that hope is within reach if they soften the way they regard themselves and alter the way they handle themselves internally and externally.

Separating depression from self-hatred can assist clients to see the eating disorder for what it is, with all its lies and implications, and assist them to start to see who they are in a more frank and precise manner.

We can extract the worldwide, ambiguous, and prospective feeling of depression and split it into narrower parts, more particular, more direct, and more mentally linked to their experiences than to their identity.

We're talking a bunch about their emotions of pain and sorrow, and exploring and deepening their knowledge of feeling unloved, or their sense of inadequacy, or their emotions of dismissal and disapproval, etc. In very particular and emotionally connected understandings and phrases, I attempt to underpin depression.

I rarely speak to them directly about their depression as we try to comprehend, validate, and build hope in particular fields of their pain.

I discovered it more useful to spend meetings discussing how to build self-esteem over a sense of failure, a sense of powerlessness, a feeling of dissatisfaction, etc., rather than speaking about depression and what to do to assist lessen it.

The result is that we are also de-amplifying and de-escalating the depression in the phase of fostering trust by concentrating on and debating the distinct types of pain. It's difficult to get to the bottom of the depression and prevent the particular pain as avoiding the pain is what clients tried to do through the eating disorder.

It is essential to remember here that DNA can and is generally engaged in the quality, severity, and form of depression they experience, and that thorough assessment and use of antidepressant drugs is highly promoted as an effective aspect of the therapy. It is also essential to note that clients with serious eating disorders often withstand drug use or sabotage as an effort to regulate their body and weight and promote a feeling of power.

It is essential to be very careful and frequently monitor the use of medication and to try to assist them in the beneficial understanding of medication use. Too often, medicine reflects vulnerability and becomes proof to participate in self-hatred again rather than being seen as yet another piece of the puzzle that will assist to build hope in their rehabilitation.

It is my view that if we can reframe the medicine as a positive aspect of their healing and rehabilitation from both depression and an eating disorder, clients often react to and profit from therapy.

It is also essential to continue assessing and recognizing the effect of malnutrition on the capacity of clients to process and/or alter the manner they handle data about themselves and their life when interacting with an eating disorder. Reducing Isolation moving them out of the difficulty is another significant element in the treatment of depression among eating disorder clients.

Often, re-engaging and reconnecting with other individuals is a very strong action for clients. Moving away from isolation and reconnecting in their life with others brings hope.

Pursuing a reconnection with others emphasizes being open to feeling linked, feeling the love, empathy, and concern of others towards them, and expressing their empathy and love towards family members, colleagues, other clients or patients, etc.

Involving couples in family therapy, couple therapy associates, and treatment buddies are often very strong methods of reducing depression and increasing customer hope because they feel comforted and endorsed by those who love and care for them.

Helping clients in their life to interact with individuals again brings hope and renewed capacity to feel something distinct from self-hatred. Receiving expressions of affection, interest, and real care of someone else is promising and becomes a very significant component of depression therapy.

Again, it is because of self-hatred that the guilt becomes special for those with eating diseases. The guilt informs them to feel bad and awful about themselves because they are not ideal, or are not in full command, or have not been achieved, or have not been adopted or liked by all, or because there are dissatisfied individuals in their life. A pain that is not going to cure is the fake guilt connected with fake or incorrect perceptions.

Working with eating disorder clients is useful in helping them understand the distinction between actual guilt and fake guilt. We can assist them to acknowledge that true guilt is linked to doing something incorrect literally. Their acknowledgment of that may guide them to correct it. False guilt informs them to feel bad and awful about themselves, and anything that has occurred is the proof against them that promotes guilty feeling.

I often attempt to assist clients to know particular methods in which fake guilt gets into the image and feeds self-hatred. It is often linked to fields of their life where they feel or feel helpless but have become mentally accountable. An example of this might be feeling bad about themselves because they feel responsible for a particular outcome of the relationship, they don't have the authority to produce themselves.

They may feel bad about themselves because they can't fix a situation or trouble experiencing someone they love or care about, or because they can't stop a disaster. False guilt is a sense of shame, a sense of "knowing better" or "figuring it out" in advance.

False guilt is often an indication of what it is not, rather than who it is or what it can do. Sometimes the fake guilt is just an effective manifestation of the intense pattern of adverse contrast that is so prevalent with eating disorders between themselves and others.

Clients with eating disorder constantly compare with someone else, both physically and behaviorally, and end up feeling a lot of guilt about who they are because they don't match up with someone else in their comparison.

False guilt is sometimes an expression of self-hatred for some wrong done in the past, something they won't let go of or excuse themselves.

They try to punish themselves constantly for what occurred or for what they feel terrible about doing, sometimes long ago. They retain it mentally as assistance for their self-rejection against themselves.

The fake guilt and feeling terrible about themselves are often immediately linked to how important people are behaving or acting in their life. They tend to feel somehow responsible or responsible for the adverse decisions or actions of someone else.

False guilt provides them a feeling of hopelessness because their capacity to alter it or re-frame it is impeded by their self-contempt filter all-around. They can compare themselves to irrational self-standards that no one could live up to, and thus become the exception to all normalcy regulations. They have to live above acceptable somehow, and the sense of guilt is evidence that they don't live at the greater stage of achievement that is anticipated.

Often when they hear input from other individuals about their habits, especially their eating disorder, feeling fake guilt becomes another incentive. The problem with self-guilt is that it produces intense feelings of fault, blame, guiltiness, shame, depression, and sadness, but instead of moving them to correction and change, it moves them to self-hatred, self-criticalness, self-doubting, and self-punishment.

False guilt always contributes to a greater lack of hope. Releasing fake guilt fosters hope because setting clear mental limits contributes to an enhanced feeling of liberty and decisions.

Until we do that, we probably won't see the scope and magnitude of depression and the very private aspect of how depression manifests itself in feeding clients with illness.

It is also essential to raise our knowledge and comprehension of how depression is unique to those suffering from eating disorders as it provides us therapy alternatives and a structure to interfere with those with these coexisting illnesses more sympathetically and optimistically. The most useful thing we can do with these clients in every meeting is to build hope.

Nurturing trust is not always a clear and clear list of methods or procedures, but a desire on the part of both client and therapist to confront the hopelessness in a kind and caring environment.

I hope these therapy differences and suggestions start to promote some hope for clients with coexisting depression and eating disorders. In confronting hopelessness, pain, self-hatred, guilt, and loneliness, we can gradually promote and build hope and reduce depression.

SECTION 2

Forms in which Depression can occur

What is the reason why the number of people who are depressed is rapidly increasing?

The World Health Organization (WHO) issued a report stating that the number of people experiencing depression doubles every 10 years and that by 2020 it will be the world's most prevalent disease and the second leading cause of death. Why is this happening in a wealthy society like ours that is currently spending more money on medical care than ever in history?

The number of people suffering from the debilitating effects of depression contributes to this increase in many factors.

This book will shed some light on some of these factors.

Our news media is a major factor contributing to the rise of depression. The news on TV, radio, and newspapers focus almost exclusively on the small percentage of things that are wrong in our world out of all the good things that happen every day.

Believing what you hear or read in the news gives you the impression that our planet's world situation and physical condition are in a downward spiral with little hope of improvement.

If you watch, listen, or read the news daily, you feed your mind with the garbage equivalent. Have you ever heard the term "garbage in, garbage out" on the computer? Not only with computers but also with the human mind.

The prescriptions for antidepressants issued to children and adolescents between 1987 and 1996 grew three to tenfold. Between 1998 and 2002, despite the lack of evidence they cure depression, there was a 50 percent overall increase in antidepressant prescriptions.

A study conducted by Express Scripts reports the April 2004 issue of the journal "Psychiatric Services." This study shows that the use of antidepressant medicines among children and adolescents continues to increase by about 10 percent annually.

U.K. And U.S. studies show that many young patients taking these drugs have increased suicidal tendencies. In their lives, children and adolescents are at a stage where their brain is rapidly developing. This raises a question about the unknown and long-term side effects prescribed by these drugs during this critical growth stage.

Although it is an option to use natural remedies, doctors rarely suggest their use. When discussing natural remedies in her book "Molecules of Emotion," Candace Pert, Ph.D. (recognized as the world's leading brain researcher) has this to say concerning natural remedies: "The answer reflects the economies of medicine.

Because the natural substances are not patentable, there is no incentive for drug companies to study their benefits, and so the vast majority of M.D.s who get the benefit of the medicine is not patentable. How are they doing that? According to Kevin Trudeau in his book "Natural Cures' They' Don't Want You To Know About,' they do it by" producing their product at the lowest possible cost, selling it at the highest price, and selling as much as they can.

"According to Mr. Trudeau," the healthcare industry, defined as the treatment, prevention, and diagnosis of disease, is the most profitable in the world. Getting healthy and staying healthy is not in the best interests of pharmaceutical companies.

Our school system still focuses pretty much on learning the three R's: reading, writing, and arithmetic. Yes, these are important basics that you need to work well in society. But to succeed in life, one needs to know more than these basics.

Have you ever studied in school for a test and passed with flying colors just to forget all the answers when it wasn't important to remember them anymore?

In one of his earlier books, "If You Want to Be Rich & Happy: Don't Go to School?: Ensuring Lifetime Security for Yourself and Your Children" published in 1995, well-known and respected financial author of the book series "Rich Dad," Robert T. Kiyosaki, touched on this topic. He believes there is a flaw in a system that rewards students for memorizing facts but does not help them to be successful in the real world.

In all subjects, a standard is set today and it is expected that every child will achieve that standard. If they don't, their teacher and the school system in general look at them as deficient in some way, or less than perfect. This comparison system is detrimental to the child's self-esteem that leads to depression.

Concern What Other People Think. People often worry about what other people, especially males, will think of them if they seek help for their depression. There is the mistaken belief that depression is something that only women have, which causes men to feel that they are "weak" when depressed.

There is also a tendency for people who are depressed to see themselves as failures and to take on the belief that others see them as failures. They end up spending a lot of energy worrying about their depression and doing little or nothing to get help.

Our Natural Tendency toward Dependency. Most of us are taught from the time we are born to rely on others to know what is best for us and tell us what to do.

We were taught to rely on our parents to know what's best for us when we're young and even adults. We were taught to look at our teachers and schools to see what would be best for us if our parents didn't know. For our spiritual needs, we were taught to rely on our preferred religious organization, on doctors and conventional medicine for our health needs, on the government to provide for and care for us after retirement (or before), etc.

This attitude has led us to believe that our lives or our destiny are not in control. This fosters impotence feelings that naturally lead to depression.

Teen depression–Work depression hormones are something that can be said to be quite common among people all over the world and in almost any situation, and depression can appear and manifest in many forms within the body. Now adolescents, or depression in adolescents, is something that can happen quite commonly in these pubescent human beings who are going through a whole host of hormonal and physical changes.

The problem here is that while some adolescents may be able to cope with these natural growth functions, some others may not be able to cope so well and show their inability to cope with things such as depression. Now when one person goes through puberty, hormonal changes are taking place in the body, and the dark thing is that hormones have so much to do with the body's emotional subsystems.

There is an increase in the amount of male or female hormones circulating the body when you grow up or experience puberty, and this is because your body is trying to activate the biological triggers within the body to start some growth spurt and allow areas within the body to grow and develop that mark you as male or female.

Now when you're a male, your body's testosterone level increases, triggering processes such as protein synthesis and male-specific organ development, and other body functions. Your Adam's apple is booming, the voice box is going to deepen, protein synthesis is going to make sure your muscularity is growing and your mass and height are going to be affected as well. The hormone we are talking about here for the female is estrogen and it performs the same functions as testosterone but affects only different areas of the female body.

Now, with any biological processes and the millions of possible genetic combinations out there, in individuals who are experiencing puberty, there are bound to be side effects and levels of side effects. One of them is that they are unable to cope with their major physical changes and may experience things like acne that could cause them to feel depressed about their appearance.

Hormones at such a level may also give rise to emotions to go up and down like tidal waves, and these teenagers may be out of control to handle.

Because of these emotions and feelings of segmentation from other normal people, they may slide into the depression that is common to adolescents. Do not be alarmed if you see your teenager, even for an extended period, showing signs of depression. Their body is trying to get used to the high hormone levels and the massive changes they are going through.

Be concerned if they become a complete introvert and in themselves, there is a drastic change of character. Then more than just the normal hormonal problem could be the problem. If you're concerned, get in touch with a child psychologist who can help you evaluate your teenager and make recommendations.

Depression in Women

There's an incredibly heartless stigma associated with depression... Especially those who never experienced it! Part of this stigma is that more than men, fairer sex often struggles with depression.

This leads to depression as a mere character defect or even a sign of weakness. There could be nothing beyond the truth. Depression is a mental disorder caused by several different circumstances and requires different levels of case-by-case treatment. There may be similar signs of depression in women, but treatment varies significantly every time. And despite the higher prevalence of depression in women, it affects both men and women.

Clinically depressed women face unimaginable challenges. It's a very serious condition that hurts her self-esteem, relationships, social life, and also work. Women's depression causes great impacts on their lives and reduces any chance of getting the best out of life and herself. It may seem hopeless without great support from her close relationships.

Does that sound grim? It is! Especially when you stop taking into account women's depression frequency. There is one in eight chances that she will suffer from a major depressive disorder, according to the National Mental Health Association, some time in a woman's life.

However, not all doom and gloom can be treated as depression in women. Treatment success depends on how well your symptoms can be identified and understood. The better you're educated about depression and the road ahead, the better you're going to get. The first step is to identify the signs.

Signs of Depression in Women

- Lack of interest in activities that are usually pleasant, including sex
- A significant decline in energy and overwhelming fatigue
- Sleeping extremes— either way too little a clink
- Difficulty making decisions or remembering basic things
- Feelings of hopelessness, helplessness, worthlessness, anger, and guilt

Signs of Depression in Women that require immediate attention.

Persistent headache and chronic pain that does not respond to medication

- constant feeling of sadness, depression, and emptiness
- excessive crying (you cry for no reason) and extreme bouts of unexplained irritability
- suicidal behavior or thoughts

Are there any more serious signs of depression in women?

Depression is significant in anybody, male or female, and should be addressed as soon as possible. While both sexes have similar signs and symptoms of depression, it is the way they consider these signs of depression themselves that makes the difference.

All components of life are viewed differently by men and women, almost opposites in fact, and the same goes for causes of depression. As an example, men look to blame others when things go wrong, while women blame themselves. As opposed to women avoiding conflict, men can also look for conflict. Men will be watching over their problems and women will be afraid of themselves meanwhile. Furthermore, in today's society, there is a great deal of social pressure for women including having children, juggling a career and having a husband, creating the perfect home, and maintaining that perfect Vogue covers girls body! It should come as no surprise with all these factors that you see signs of depression more frequently in women than in men!

A major sign of Women's Depression - Negativity and self-loathing

Despite the source, steady negativity is not just a type of personality but one of the noticeable signs of women's depression.

It could be anything from poor body image, poor financial positioning, or some other stress forming situations at home, at work, or social. Too often women are tagged as a negative bellyacher or whinger, but the truth is that once depression takes hold, it all looks dark and hopeless, and no way out appears. Even in fundamental situations.

The key is to recognize your depression, causes, triggers, and clarify what you need to get right again. Treatments vary from woman to woman and are related to symptoms. Anywhere from natural depression cures to hormone replacement therapy, prescription medication, conventional therapy, regular exercises, and cleaning up your diet can help and it can be surprisingly effective even to get out in the sun!

Helping friends, family, your partner, and your family physician as soon as you first begin to see the signs of depression in women is of critical importance. Don't wait too long for help as it counts every single day!

Depression is an awful condition, and with an incredibly cruel stigma attached to it, it is sadly completely misunderstood. Information is key with this type of disease and the more we know about the symptoms and triggers of depression, the better we are to deal with it.

Postpartum Depression

Postpartum Depression is a mixture of changes in physical, emotional, and behavior that occur after a woman's birth or miscarriage. This type of depression takes place for about four weeks after delivery. The "baby blues" occurs for the first few weeks after the birth. Baby blues usually go away in a couple of weeks, but post-partum depression may last for months.

Baby blues signs: Sleeping disorder Feeling moody Teary Feeling overwhelmed sleeping disorder Mixed feelings of being happy about your baby Any woman may experience post-partum depression in months after birth, stillbirth, or miscarriage.

Bio-identical progesterone drugs with side effects

The sooner you receive treatment, the sooner you feel better and enjoy your baby. You can make an informed choice.

Are you at risk?

Postpartum risk factors for depression are:

- your pregnancy age
- the younger you are, the higher the risk if you have ambivalent feelings of pregnancy from your partner, friends, family, or living alone. What are the signs of postpartum depression? Before the number of children you have had depression
- the more you have, the more likely you have had previous depressions.

Common signs of depression are:

- A feeling that is very sad, worthless, hopeless, anxious, and empty.
- Loss of enjoyment in everyday things.
- Do not feel hungry and in the opposite direction, you may lose weight or weight and gain weight.
- Can't be concentrated.
- Death thoughts
- Mood changes
- Energy or tiredness

What causes it?

After birth, postpartum depression is associated with hormone changes. After delivery, the changes involve a rapid drop in estrogen and progesterone hormones. The problem with these symptoms is that estrogen production occurs much more quickly while progesterone remains at a very low level.

Hormones for a healthy pregnancy - estrogen and progesterone

The hormones of estrogen and progesterone during pregnancy are the two most important hormones. They help the breasts increase the fetus ' milk uterus, the placenta supports the baby, and the immune system would not be slightly suppressed to prevent the baby from attacking. Only progesterone is produced during pregnancy until the baby is born. The term pro-gestation originated from the hormone of progesterone.

The new mother has to adjust to the new progesterone and estrogen levels after delivery, which falls to almost zero after birth. Natural progesterone is an antidepressant that enhances the function of the thyroid.

Estrogen and progesterone regulate vital functions of the body, are supposed to counterbalance one another, to keep you balanced, healthy, and without symptoms of postpartum depression. If your body no longer balances progesterone and opposes estrogen...

Then the hormonal environment is dominated by estrogen. It may be TOXIC for unbalanced estrogen! Symptoms of estrogen dominance, postpartum depression, postpartum psychosis, and symptoms of postpartum depression will be experienced.

The bio-identical natural choice of Progesterone for depression experienced after childbirth According to late Dr. John R. Lee, postpartum depression symptoms can be effectively treated by bio-identical progesterone cream. "It could make it much easier to deal with postpartum depression." Natural progesterone cream contains bio-identical molecules that imitate the natural progesterone of a woman. It's the same as the progesterone produced by your body. Instant results have been seen in many patients using natural progesterone cream. A woman needs to understand that natural choices can ease her symptoms. A woman can begin with natural progesterone cream by knowing and understanding her hormonal fluctuations. Progesterone balances the low or high or low progesterone ratio. Natural cream of progesterone is the only bio-identical hormone that can effectively relieve your symptoms.

Wild Yam and Chaste Tree Berry Natural Progesterone Cream is a natural choice. Healthcare professionals and women who want natural support to conceive are very popular with it.

Natural cream of progesterone treats at its source post-partum depression. It is the only natural remedy addressing the cause of the imbalance in hormones. The cause of hormone imbalance is the estrogen-progesterone ratio and all hormones decrease.

How to Prevent Post - Partum Depression Using Positivity

A growing number of women are now seeing the reality behind the postpartum depression concept for themselves. Research shows that, after giving birth, 10 percent of women experience major postpartum depression, and this has had lasting effects on them.

At about 30 to 80 percent, a higher percentage experiences a certain level of depression that, although mild, still affects their self-esteem and state of mind.

Postpartum depression is usually accompanied by a lot of weeping, tiredness, mood swings, and irritability. Many factors such as hormonal changes have been attributed to it. It can last between a few hours and a few weeks anywhere, although in some women it happens longer. Some women had to look for treatment such as a drug or therapy, or both, just to get past this difficult stage.

But the time after birth is an incredible stage in the life of a woman. Depression shouldn't accompany it. If you want to keep the depression of the post-partum at bay or at least at a minimum, all you need is:

"Me" hour. Some women say that postpartum depression is accompanied by thoughts about the sacrifices you've made and are expected to make now that you're a new mother because of the major change in your life. So, it's important to not forget about yourself and your needs after pregnancy, even in the frenzy that your new baby is causing.

Take as much time as you can for yourself, regardless of whether you're taking a bath in the bathroom for just a few extra minutes.

You can still pamper yourself and take care of your body this way. Since self-esteem is one of the first to go in the face of post-partum depression, having the time to take care of your body and doing so can help a lot as it makes you feel you are still taking care of yourself and you have not let go.

Self-care-from the beginning of your pregnancy - a plan for you. Most unplanned pregnancies are more likely to be followed by postpartum depression because before pregnancy the new mother had no set plan for herself. There are many unforeseen things to prepare for after pregnancy, and when a new mom isn't fully prepared for them, postpartum depression has an easier way to get in.

So, while you're pregnant, plan how to take care of yourself, both during pregnancy and after it. Don't let go and don't use your pregnancy as an excuse to look crappy and bloated. Look for ways to address common pregnancy issues and do something about them. For example, there is no reason to gain excess weight that you cannot get off after you give birth; this is due to poor eating choices and lifestyle choices during pregnancy.

Your self-care plan should include: a nutritional plan A rest/sleep plan A body/skincare plan A weight plan This way, you know how to deal with the changes that may occur in you and your body, and you will be prepared to deal with them.

Good thoughts. Most importantly, the power of positive thoughts is needed. There is a frightening number of destructive thoughts that after giving birth can bother a vulnerable you. But if you keep your mind focused on positive thoughts, it will resist these destructive thoughts more strongly. This way, you won't get a free pass into your life after Partum depression.

By sending subliminal messages directly to your subconscious mind, you can fill your head with positive thoughts. This way, no matter what negativity your conscious mind tries to enter your life, it won't penetrate because your subconscious has been programmed to always look at the bright side of things that will now revolve around your new baby, which is another reason for you to live positively.

Fish oil Supplement Can Protect You from Post-Partum Depression

Are you aware that one in ten women is suffering from postpartum depression? This is a terrible mental condition after giving birth that affects women. It's a serious issue as a woman with this condition is a threat to herself and her baby. Studies on fish oil and post-partum depression, however, show that regular intake of fish oil supplements during pregnancy reduces disease risk.

So, how does the fish oil / postpartum depression relationship work? Studies have linked this mental condition to low DHA levels; it is important to note that fish oil is DHA omega 3's best source. DHA is an important building block of the brain of the fetus; in fact, 30% of the human brain consists of DHA. Studies also show, not only that, that DHA plays a major role in the overall fetus development.

To put it another way, the fetus draws and depletes the DHA of the mother; therefore, if the mother does not replace the depleted

DHA with a regular intake of fish oil supplements, she will most likely suffer from post-partum depression.

Fish oil and post-partum depression indeed have a beneficial relationship; however, you need to be very careful when buying your supplements. Due to the polluted waters in which they live, fish contain toxic substances such as mercury and pesticides. So, make sure the supplements are distilled molecularly; this is the only method of purification that removes the toxins from the oil effectively.

You should also ensure that the supplements contain a high amount of DHA; because it is easier to concentrate, most brands on the market contain more EPA. It is recommended, however, that the amount of DHA be approximately twice the amount of EPA. The recommended minimum amount of DHA per capsule of 1000 mg fish oil is 250 mg.

Now that you know the link between fish oil and post-partum depression, I hope you'll take advantage of it from now on and protect yourself from the dreaded disease.

Does the Male Depression manifest in Women Same Way?

While women tend to get more attention when it comes to mood disorders, male depression is quite common and needs to be addressed similarly. Studies show that men are more likely to develop suicidal thoughts, and as such, learning how to best treat their depression is important.

Treating male depression is slightly different from treating women, although it is possible to use many of the same drugs or supplements. Since the root problem is usually one of feeling insufficient for men, alternatives to therapy will be different, as well as problem-solving.

We need to first identify the symptoms to treat male depression. In many cases, these are different from female symptoms. Having casual sex, over-indulging in alcohol and drugs, or taking part in other reckless behaviors, men are more likely to act out.

They will also tend to hide more from their depression because they feel it will mark them as a sign of weakness.

It is essential to recognize the symptoms of male depression as men tend to plan and commit suicide much more frequently than women. Men also tend not to advertise their suicide intentions until they are in the act, so it is extremely important to recognize depression before it reaches this point.

The man should be treated immediately after the symptoms of male depression have been identified. Going to a physician or therapist is often low on the priority list of the man. He may prefer to go online and talk in anonymous chat rooms and forums with others struggling with depression.

There are a variety of antidepressants on the market such as Prozac, Zoloft, and Norpramin, but men may prefer natural methods of treating depression, including herbal supplements, due to the stigma and weakness attached to the disease.

Nobody asks about the use of Ginkgo Biloba, it is a well-known enhancer of memory and clarity. Chamomile relieves stress as well as soothes and men may feel more comfortable taking it than a prescription drug that may raise questions.

Men may also be concerned that they may suffer repercussions at work and in the community if they take a prescription antidepressant or seek therapy for their problem. This is another reason that many choose to go with supplements, particularly folic acid and other B vitamins that have proven track records to reduce symptoms of depression.

Other alternative ways to treat male depression include changing the diet to include a vitamin and mineral balance, getting enough sleep, and taking steps to reduce stress at work and home. Also, daily exercise can help.

Depression is not yet fully understood in men. Many men are suspected to hide their depression successfully, so estimates of 6 million affected in the U.S. may be grossly below the true number of men affected by this disease.

Postpartum Depression in Fathers

Any mother can picture the first moment they bring into the world their newborn and the amazing experience of taking the newborn home along with all the changes and responsibilities of becoming a new mother. Postpartum depression, based on a variety of reports, affects new mothers up to 70 percent to 80 percent over the first week of giving birth and quickly passes away in some cases.

There is almost 13 percent of moms suffer from postpartum depression at the clinical level, which lasts longer periods.

The reality is that this is a normal condition produced by rapid hormonal fluctuations and changes in parenthood for countless women, but did you realize that postpartum depression can also occur in males? How many males can pick up this disease if this is the situation?

While there have been many explorations of women's condition, postpartum depression affecting males is a factual incident and more frequent than anybody would ever have known. Postpartum depression in males ranges from 10% to more or less 25% based on several kinds of research made, which makes it clear as bad if not worse than in females.

Because postpartum depression is a disease that has received little interest in males, there are fewer places where males can turn to for help. Another known fact is that if males feel signs of postpartum depression, they are also less likely to talk about their illness as voluntarily as women would, and more often less willing to ask about professional assistance.

This is the basis of the most possible rationale because males would feel disadvantaged when they present their weakness and may be embarrassed by the disease, leading to the disease not being treated and the disease becoming worse.

Causes. Some studies conducted between 1980 and 2009 yielded some fascinating results showing that approximately a quarter of the males examined developed depression within three to six months. Surprisingly, some of the victims were fathers for the first time. It has been hypothesized that because of the many adjustments and anxieties of their new parenting position, the rationale most first-time fathers pick up this condition.

It was also noted that both conditions of parents could directly affect the others and trigger depression for the first-time father if the woman has postpartum depression. At this time, the reasons for postpartum depression affecting first-time fathers are mostly speculative, although investigations have been carried out as far back as 1980, the origin of the disease in first-time fathers has not been investigated in depth.

Symptoms. Signs of disease are similar to women in first-time fathers, but there are distinct differences. Women would usually feel worthlessness, sorrow, and depression, and more often than not, so do fathers of the first time, but distinct differences consist of translating feelings of sorrow into abandonment, anger, and touch. Although these signs have been observed, the results are still unsettled and more research is needed to understand it in this area. Postpartum depression is a terrible disease in first-time fathers and can ruin the family relationship with both the younger and the mother more often than not. First-time fathers should genuinely recognize their illness and not be afraid to immediately try to find treatment alternatives.

Identification and treatment. As discussed earlier, fathers for the first time tend to be more ignorant of the disease than mothers who can discuss their disease without reservation. Because this is the case, the woman or other family members should be responsible for identifying the signs of the disease and discussing the disease with the man and making him aware of the disease.

He should be open to treatment once he acknowledges the disease and should talk to his doctor who can point him to the appropriate treatment path. Postpartum depression treatment may include psychiatric and drug therapy or a combination of both. The sooner you try to find treatment, the sooner you can get to a speedy recovery and help you with your family on your way to a normal happy life.

Strategies to Beat Male Depression

Male depression is often hidden because men are not as expressive as women about their emotions. However, men who are depressed and succeed in keeping the world hidden are often prone to sudden violent outbursts. The main cause of men beating their wives or abusing their children is male depression. These traits make learning some basic strategies for beating male depression critical for all men.

It is important to know that there are two different causes of male depression. Depression in males is often the result of some childhood traumatic experience. Oddly enough, this is often caused by witnessing his father beating his mother or abusing himself. It's not known the other cause. There is no apparent reason for depression to develop.

The first key to beating it, regardless of the cause of the depression, is to realize that the depression exists and is a problem.

Men who are covered, hidden, depressed are usually reluctant to seek help. Generally speaking, it takes something very drastic to happen to make a man realize that he has a big problem that requires treatment, such as his wife leaving him.

Once a man realizes he's having a depression problem, he can start looking for treatment. His family and friends ' medicines, therapy, and support can go a long way towards curing depression.

The man must take the final step by changing his life outlook and realizing that no one else can make him happy. He has to accept life, like it or not, and he's the only one that can make him happy.

It's possible to beat male depression. The steps of treating a woman for depression are the same. The main difference is the key step of making the man realize he's ill, but there's the treatment that can cure him if he's willing to accept help and make an effort on his own.

Differences Between Men and Women Depression Recovery Process

Depression affects far fewer men than women, yet on a global scale, it is a six percent figure. Although the drugs and treatment offered to women with depression are similar to those offered to men, there are different symptoms. Therefore, recovery of male depression must be approached differently.

Men react differently compared to women in terms of dealing with depression, according to the majority of physicians and therapists. Men are more inclined to anger, misery, and violence. Males are more likely to lose their self-control while women experience higher levels of insignificant and hopeless feelings.

Many of the signs, however, are common to men and women alike. Some of the most common signs and symptoms include:

- feelings of sorrow
- feelings of worthlessness for no obvious reason
- sudden weight loss
- appetite changes
- putting on weight
- eating too much
- not being able to sleep
- feeling irritated
- lower energy levels
- often feeling drained and sleepy
- often feeling guilty for no apparent reason
- unexplained ache

While women find their grief easier to verbalize and are more likely to shed tears. They are also more likely to increase their number of sleeping hours and sometimes eat too much, even though men still go to work more frequently, visit the gym and continue their daily commitments.

Males also tend not to tell their family and friends how they feel, but to keep their thoughts to themselves. When this happens, they usually break away from their normal social life, which tends to make matters worse, and is one of the many reasons why male depression can be hard to discover.

Although many treatments and medicines are readily available to help men recover from depression, encouraging them to ask for such remedies or even simply see a doctor is often rather challenging. This is when the worst becomes their condition.

If you know someone who is going through depression, try talking to them to see a professional so that they can get the medication they need.

Make sure you give extra care and support to them. If you see that they experience frustration and other signs and symptoms associated with men's depression, try reaching out to them and giving them a helping hand. To help them better understand their condition, you could give them some books or extra materials.

These resources may even persuade them to seek professional help.

Remember that this condition is easier to handle at an early stage plus the fact that it is possible to start their recovery from depression the sooner they can be supported.

Depression & Andropause-How to Help Yourself

Andropause is directly correlated with depression-a major player-facing men in their late 40s to late 50s in the notorious mid-life crisis period. During this mid-life transition, hormone-wrecked men experience a wide variety of symptoms and conditions-everything from mental (i.e. irritability) to physical (loss of libido, lack of energy, and weight gain.) Depression, left untreated, can be a disabling condition.

Andropause depression is caused by lowering testosterone levels. Low levels of testosterone cause many depressive symptoms-including a general indifference to your surrounding events, inability to concentrate, extreme irritability, and memory loss.

We could stress things in a normal situation that might otherwise be worry-free and brood over certain matters. Our memory may go down the drain and we may start seeing our lives in a negative light.

The levels of energy collapse and enthusiasm for the activities we used to enjoy becoming flat-lined. Another common symptom is insomnia and restlessness. Normal things could become a burden for us, and a child's simplest cry can make us overly irritable.

Psychologists use a variety of battery tests to determine if you have depression. They also place you under observation in addition to handing you test sheets to work with-noticing your behavior, tendencies, and habits while talking to them.

Men tend to be by nature rebellious creatures. We love to shrug our faults off and stand during an emotional disturbance.

We assume the role of masculine creatures-jungle lion kings who reign over the widespread landscape we call life. When it comes to questions about their sexual ability and prowess, men can be in complete denial. Refusing to understand that, as a result of Andropause, we are not in our blood who we once were with our sexual performance.

Fellas, it's time to get to know the severity of your depression.

Off the bat, as a major problem, some facts and figures support depression. For one, men perform 80 percent of all suicides in the U.S. Most people with this condition never seek therapists, psychologists, and psychiatrists ' advice and counsel.

Probably the most shocking fact of all is that during the Andropause years the male suicide rate is the highest. You are reading correctly-the highest in the years we're talking about specifically.

How are we going to handle these devastating changes in our lives? How can the chances of clinical depression be reduced by managing stress? We have to follow a daily exercise scheme for one. That combined with a caffeine-free diet will boost our disease-fighting immune systems. It will also slow the process of aging. Aim to keep the 30-inch, vertical, explosive leap into your 60s! Another is doing the things we love. Do not stray from playing your basketball pick-up games with buddies or from scratch as a hobby building those go-carts. Stick to them and enjoy doing so with pleasure. Distract yourself from your current state without completely ignoring it.

Maintain a friendly and family social network that will cheer you when you need it most. Something as simple as having your kid shoot a hand drawing in your face of a red school bus can make you smile and laugh. The most important piece of advice is to accept and make the best of your condition.

For example, low testosterone levels with testosterone cream can be easily supplemented. It's bound to happen to us all, and you can either make the best of it or let it overwhelm you. Consciousness is critical, and an optimistic attitude, followed by physical activity and a solid nutritional plan, is the best way to combat Andropause, anti-aging, and the demon known as depression.

Depression-Suicide and Sex

While women seem to attract media attention as a gender, men are in crisis and little is talked about. If you visit sites such as the National Institute of Mental Health and the Mayo Clinic, they will report that men are less likely to suffer from women's depression.

However, the unspoken piece is the apparent disconnect between the rates of depression and the fact that men are four times more likely than women to commit suicide. Let me tell you the happy and happy man is NOT thinking about ending his life. This is not just a U.S. problem for recording. The Australian Health and Welfare Institute report using the figures from 2003-04 indicates that although suicide is declining in Oz, 79 percent of victims are male.

The report also said that 30-34-year-old men and the highest risk are then one of diagnosis and identification at nearly five times the suicide rate. In both professional sites, men are less likely to admit to depression and it is less likely to be suspected by doctors.

However, in women, symptoms are identified and diagnosed twice as frequently as men as depression. The reason for this is women's apparent ability to be more connected with their feelings, while men are working to preserve a powerful image.

So literally men are dying because they can not express themselves properly. Here are a few more surprising pieces of information from the WISQARS System 1 Centers for Disease Control and Prevention.

1. Suicide was the eighth leading cause of male death and the seventeenth leading cause of female death in 2004. Men die four times the rate of women by suicide.
2. In suicide attempts, men use more lethal methods.
3. Women are more likely to attempt suicide but are not successful primarily because of their method choice. (Pills, and so on)
4. In the 15-19 age group, nearly four times as many men as women died of suicide.
5. In the 20-24 age group, more than six times as many men as women died of suicide
6. Non-Hispanic white men aged 85 or older are at an even higher risk of suicide than anyone else in society.

The ongoing risk factors for attempts at non-fatal suicide are usually addiction, divorce or depression, and/or other mental disorders. TAKE IT SERIOUSLY if you or anyone you know has expressed thoughts about suicide. The most important thing is the last scary piece of information about suicide in depression and the sexes.

1. Women tend to take a relatively long time to attempt the initial thoughts of suicide. This time frame may be as long as 42 months or 3.5 years, some research has indicated.

2.   Men take a much shorter time from initial suicide expression to attempting the act to think through their plans. This time frame is about 12-14 months or just over a year somewhere.

Given male suicide's lethal tools of choice and the higher rate of taking their own lives successfully, and this compressed "consideration time" is indeed a serious issue.

Most attempts to commit suicide are expressions of extreme distress, not harmless attention bids. A person who seems suicidal should not be left alone and should receive immediate treatment for mental health.

SECTION 3

Effective Strategies to Combat Depression

Depression is one of people's most worrying and chronic illnesses.

This takes place in all age groups irrespective of whether you are a child, old age, middle age, or teenager. The incidence rate is 1 out of 5 individuals. Women are more vulnerable to depression than males, and there is no particular reason for it to happen.

It is suspected, though, that it has something to do with chemical brain imbalances. The most common symptoms include depression, worthlessness, hopelessness, helplessness, feelings of guilt, tiredness, sleeping difficulties, frustration, and negative thoughts that may contribute to suicide attempts by the sufferer.

It is a condition that can be treated and you can combat it quite quickly.

Citizens were healed by more than 80 million. If you want to battle this then with the aid of professionals you need to follow the proper methods of treatment.

Usually, people depend on the form of treatment to combat depression, medications and antidepressants are used. Such antidepressant drugs contain side effects, but patients are still searching for those methods of treatment that do not cause side effects. Here are some of the best non-drug methods:

1.   The best and most effective approach is through psychotherapy. Therapies such as cognitive behavioral therapy, group therapy, and family therapy are the best methods for treatment to recognize depression symptoms that impact the client. Suitable help is given by finding the signs in the sufferer that a sufferer has something that is missing. Another form of psychotherapy called speech therapy is helpful for teaching methods of treating depression by recognizing

the root cause in the client. Depressed people found themselves happier and understood more about their lives. People don't consider talking to a psychologist yet, they feel ashamed or embarrassed, but they have to know that this is the best way to overcome this challenge.

2. Regular workout in the gym or at home can allow you to blast all the bad energy in the form of sweatiness. You're going to be comfortable and renewed.

3. Go for a weekend film and enjoy yourself.

4. Become socially active, partake in social activities, seek to engage in some social activities, do so would include you in social activities and there will be no space for depression.

5. Have someone to speak to share your feelings, you can have yourself happy and comfortable when sharing your feelings.

6. Good sleep has something to do with it as well, make sure you sleep properly.

In the battle against depression, a balanced diet often plays a major role. Make sure you have a healthy diet. Do not take too much alcohol because it includes depressants. Alcohol frequently causes severe depression.

Best Medication for Depression - Supplements, Meditation, and Psychotherapy

While antidepressants have been effective in treating depression and anxiety, due to side effects, a large number of people suffering from these conditions are not coping well and are getting worse than ever with these drugs. Most psychologists, doctors, or counselors agree vitamins, exercise or psychotherapy may be the best drug for stress and depression.

Supplements for a stable mind

The best cure for depression and anxiety is to eat healthy and well. Below is a sample of some of the products that can assist in hormone dysfunction regulation:

Turkey's cheese and food. They're high in 5-HTP amino acids. This amino acid facilitates natural serotonin production, the chemical which transmits signals in the brain between neurons. If the brain did not have this drug, the interaction would slow down and the other parts of the brain would immediately react by producing excessive amounts of hormones, resulting in hormonal imbalance.

Nevertheless, it does not mean that your daily diet must consist of turkey and cheese morning, noon, and night. You could consume certain foods and just pop a substitute for the gel capsule to preserve and increase the body's 5-HT amount. Ask your doctor about an extra 5-HT and how to prescribe it.

Liver. The liver has a high vitamin B12 content. Depressed people in their body have insufficient levels of vitamin B6 and B12. That's why most individuals with mood disorders talk of hand numbing, tremors, and sleeping difficulties. Often contained in tablets are vitamin B6 and B12. Over the counter, you can buy a bottle of them. The best way to help you sleep easily is to take this medicine at night because it relaxes the nerves.

Fish oils. The fish's head and belly are high with Omega-3. Research shows that Omega-3 helps remove a depressed person's negative and pessimistic feelings.

Meditation, 15 minutes a day

Most depressed patients feel that stress won't last long or they won't fall into despair if they only learned how to stay still and calm their heads for five minutes.

Psychiatrists approval. A patient can get through anxiety and depression without medicine for just 15 minutes a day. Meditation is probably one if not the best depression medication and stress for them. By leading the brain to calm down and think nothing but to relax, it helps to relieve pressure.

What separates relaxation from sleep is that a meditating person feels comfortable, peaceful, and refreshed even while awake. And this is what he wants through episodes of anxiety and depression: to handle his feelings and have total control over his life.

Psychotherapy. Letting everything out A therapist will help you to understand the root cause of your anxiety and depression. Thinking about the issues, activities, and situations that render you nervous, agitated, and depressed is one of the better depression anxiety therapies. You'll know how to attack them because you know what makes the thought go haywire.

You will have the opportunity to voice out everything inside your heart during a psychotherapy session. It will rid you of stress and anxiety by removing and taking out excess baggage. What's more, you can ask a therapist for guidance on how to respond to certain situations and how to control your feelings if you encounter something you're scared of.

Psychotherapy has greatly benefited the most depressed and anxious individuals. The explanation they're able to share their deepest feelings with someone they believe isn't emotionally connected to them, others claim, and thus offering them an impartial or unprejudiced opinion they can't get from family or friends.

Therefore, all that stops those two conditions from developing is the best medication for depression and anxiety. Drink vitamins, meditate and consult a therapist for psychotherapy appointments even before stress and depression hits.

Natural Home Remedies for Depression

Depression is a very dangerous disease; as soon as possible, you will try to treat it. Patients feel in despair that no one can comprehend or support them. The symptoms of depression include weight loss and benefit, hopelessness, anxiety, exhaustion, sleep off, suicide feelings and suicidal impulses, and less focus.

Because of many biological causes including menstrual cycle, abortion, infertility, premenstrual disorder, and menopause, it is more common in women.

Many individuals with distress do not receive medical care, although most patients do respond to medication. It is very important to treat depression because it also affects your life and your job. Depression is a disease that can be healed. By home remedies, natural remedies, medications, physician recommendations, etc., it can heal.

Treatment requires a mix of medical care, drug therapy, help for the community, compassion, gratitude, natural interaction, and home remedies. There are home treatments you can use for depression. Most people prefer home remedies over conventional treatments because they are healthy and have no side effects.

A natural herb is St. John's Wort. Home remedies for depression are very successful. This herb can be sold in any pharmacy or food shop. It has been used as a mood stabilizer for decades and is routinely used by many people to fight off depression or anxiety bouts.

To get rid of depression, take a candida diet. The candida triggers this. This diet will help cure the disease of depression. Candida diet includes high fiber foods and low starch vegetables such as lettuce, radish, celery, and asparagus.

Take a bath in the water. Sunlight has an element needed to balance our moods. Interact with colleagues, members of your family, play games, and do stuff you like to do.

Exercise and meditation are some of the best home treatments in treating depression. In physical movement, exercise, and yoga help, particularly repeated motion. Physical movement has been linked with promoting the synthesis and release of chemicals enhancing emotions including the serotonin neurotransmitter, which has been shown to have beneficial effects in depression.

Exercise and meditation both tend to increase levels of serotonin.

Disclaimer: This book is not meant to provide health advice and is only intended for general information. Until embarking on any health program, please try the advice of a trained health professional.

Yoga for Depression: How to Enhance Your Mental Health Through Gentle Stretching

It is well known that yoga has numerous health benefits and is often prescribed for physical ailments such as back pain, but it is interesting to explore the use of ancient methods to enhance mental well-being and provide a positive outlook on life.

New U.S. research found that three hours of gentle yoga a week can help fight depression as it increases levels of a chemical in the brain that is necessary for a calm mind. In 2010, researchers at the Boston University School of Medicine reported that amino acid GABA rates in people performing yoga were significantly higher than those doing the equivalent of a moderately strenuous exercise, such as running. These chemicals are important for brain and central nervous system work and facilitate a state of relaxation in the body.

Specific anxiety disorders and depression are associated with low rates of GABA. This would then indicate that there is more to the way yoga makes us feel happy and relaxed than just releasing endorphins like another workout.

Stress is a common occurrence in today's society; issues like the recent credit crunch and job market, in addition to raising a family, marriages, research, etc., may take us all toll. Our bodies and minds are not designed to handle long periods of pressure that can result in diabetes, obesity, skin problems, asthma, ulcers, and as described above; anxiety and depression.

How to Reduce Depression and Stress Through Focused Breathing and Understanding

Yoga provides good outcomes for depression and stress management— it reduces stress and tension through relaxing or bending into various postures (referred to as' Asanas' in yoga) and unwinds knots in back and neck muscles etc. that can cause the body to feel tight.

Physical workouts produce endorphins, natural chemicals that create a sense of well-being in the body.

Breathing exercises (called' Pranayamas') make a person take deeper breaths that flood the body with more oxygen and control blood pressure, but also be mindful of your breathing regulation is a very effective tool in the battle against stress.

-Pranayamas and Asanas, the' culture of the mind' together allow us to get to know our innermost being and to regulate ourselves through learning to control our bodies. Practitioning yoga can help you understand that there is an interconnection between brain, body, and spirit that in effect helps to maintain balance in everyday life.

-Yoga clears the mind: our brains are always moving in the transition from one idea to the next! The focus used for Asanas and Pranayamas in yoga offers the mind a well-deserved break, side by side with all other worries and emotions.

The theory also plays an important role in keeping the view more positive. Regular yoga practice may change a person's view of the world and their mindset toward achieving goals and accomplishment rather than disappointment. Asanas and Pranayamas give positive thought.

At the end of each yoga session relaxing with the' savasana' or corpse pose may feel like an unwanted relief at first but gradually becomes a total liberation for both body and mind, bringing you back into the world refreshed and ready to go!

Some main yoga postures, or asanas, are' savasana ' (corpse pose) as stated above,' balasana' (child pose),' makarasana' (crocodile pose), and' vrikshasana' (tree pose) to alleviate stress. Each time you feel stressed out, take a breather, and see how much yoga makes a difference to your attitude!

Teachers in yoga also experiment with methods to help their students deal with a variety of conditions. Depression is extreme and one of many illnesses, but it can be the "root cause" of many more difficulties, much like anxiety. Now, let's look at ten ways to turn back from depression in the life of a yoga instructor.

Severe depression situations also require professional guidance. It is, therefore, best to guide any students of Yoga in that direction, but we all have our "dark moments," so these are remedies to milder depression situations.

Meditate through Visualization and Affirmation: Also support your students in their meditation practice to be self-sufficient while you give yoga classes. Many yoga teachers have chosen forms of mindfulness, but for all yoga students to understand and practice, imagination, and encouragement are simple methods.

Students of yoga should strive to visualize something that brings them immense pleasure and does not hurt others. This is often something they can imagine very quickly. It might be a loved one, a vacation place, or a target achieved. The yoga student learns to achieve his or her dream in this training.

Affirmation is a tool that can be directed by any yoga teacher. It builds self-esteem and positive energy. There are many affirmations CDs to choose from, and we're bringing them to play with at home in the pro-shop for yoga classes. Those two approaches make productive use of alone space, and the brain, body, and soul can remove depression.

Relaxation techniques: demonstrate a range of relaxing approaches to your meditation learners. We are all acquainted with relaxation techniques on a stage-by-stage basis, but there are many more strategies to learn. Self-hypnosis DVDs often contain controlled forms of calming. For bedtime and quiet time, these are good.

Walking Time: Many of us can choose to do Sun Salutations, but like anyone else, students of Yoga may benefit from a stroll. This could be every aspect of the day; it's going to help before school, dinner, after work, or on holidays. The fresh air is a regular drudgery break that is required. Strategic exercise use to split the day has enormous health benefits.

Sleeping patterns: Going to bed earlier can help students of Yoga or anyone else get the maximum amount of sleep they can. This will also give them the next day a positive start. Students of yoga who leave the day early will have space and energy to see the sunrise for all of the above remedies.

The following morning, after a good night's sleep, sun greetings and mindfulness will keep depression "at bay." Yoga students who continue with these approaches will charge themselves emotionally and experience the force of self-empowerment.

If you know, somebody can feel very discouraged now and then-students of yoga are no different. Four further methods are available here to support yoga participants with minor forms of depression.

Stay away from being self-centered: there's no need to separate ourselves; we're linked to everything, men, nature, the cosmos, and Allah. We must be in peace with our lives and with all things we come into contact with.

Consider what you can do in a day and sleep the remainder. Once our days are over, the world must continue to run, so let the universe think about it. Stop thinking of "I" and you'll have far fewer responsibilities to bear around.

Set goals: Without ambitions, life wouldn't mean anything, so write them down and pursue them. Such aims that are morally sound and produce satisfaction should be "heartfelt." That one remedy stops most yoga students most of the time from experiencing depression.

Look at what you've always earned and don't think about what you don't have. A rich man who is concerned about what he has not is living in poverty created by himself. His money may be placed on something good, but he stays committed to protecting his resources and investment issues.

It's a shame, but it's not an isolated case. The poor struggle to find happiness, family, and friendships that are satisfying. And, "be careful what you want." Food: The truth is that food promotes life and can lead to death as well. When I was about nine years old, one of my educators found this out to me. At first, my response was incredible, but then the truth sunk in. Many people deny nutrition, and this is clear from the malnutrition that affects us. The waistline must be constantly monitored through puberty.

Yoga students must stick to a sattvic diet to keep it simple. Put limits on ethanol, caffeine, and sugars. There are occasions when most of us feel poor but are still mindful of what we are eating and drinking.

Naturally, the liquid should be drunk at all times in equal amounts. Eight glasses of quality water per day will support the body, metabolism, detox, bones, vital organs, and more. Water use will often bring a youthful appearance to your hair. Isn't that why we practice meditation, too?

Put ideas into action: Procrastination may produce some poor results in and of itself. Setting targets or writing them down has been discussed earlier, but without bringing the plans into action, such moves are meaningless.

Truly depressed is the "dreamer" who comes up with a great concept and sees someone else bring to motion a similar idea. Sometimes on the other side of the Earth, great ideas are being experimented on, and it's just a case of who brings the concept first into practice.

Coworkers and managers will also be happy to take the blame for your proposals. So, don't waste time or in any way procrastinate. Use it to your benefit when you make a mistake or learn from it, but don't "pick on a thought." The final point to discuss on this subject is how often we evaluate ourselves negatively. I always discuss the "non-judgment" of others in my yoga classes, but in this life, we are our own biggest critics. Nobody else will ever be as cruel to oneself as we can be. Until the end, stop criticizing your proposals and put them into action.

Pranayama: Clear knowledge of breath alone can help alleviate anxiety and depression. Pranayama can be a powerful tool if you pair this with mindfulness. They know a lot about yogic breathing methods as a yoga practitioner, but students should have a few "go-to" everyday coping strategies for pranayama and some for severe stress.

The first choice would be Ujjayi Pranayama; it implies "victory and triumphant wind" translated into English. Thus, it is no surprise that this specific Pranayama purges depression and internal fears. Ujjayi Pranayama should trust as a matter of fact.

When students of yoga perform Ujjayi Pranayama with an Asana sequence including Sun Salutations or a set of Vinyasa, they can overcome mild depression and develop new self-confidence.

There are many more Yogic approaches for anybody to get rid of anxiety and gain self-confidence, but Yoga teachers and most yoga students are acquainted with these ten techniques. It is necessary to take yoga practice home, just like homework. If a student of yoga truly needs to see progress, the practice of yoga must be consistently practiced.

There are many dimensions inside yoga, but they all lead to good health. A practitioner of yoga who exercises "once in a while" is better off than not exercising at all, but should not expect significant effects to be seen. This is why instructors of yoga have to tell the truth regarding aspirations to their pupils.

Do not take the responsibility of a yoga instructor to perform yoga on an almost daily basis "sugar coat." This is also how medication for drugs operates. Could you imagine what would happen if patients once in a while are avoiding their prescribed medicine?

Continuity is the key to good wellbeing and good mental, physical, and spiritual wellness can come from a consistent yoga practice. This also refers to all that is worth doing in general.

Yoga Depression Postures

A person with depression may regularly feel depressed, unhappy, nervous, and irritated. There are many types of depression treatment and a prudent leap forward in the quest for professional counseling (psychotherapy). To help people deal with depression, support groups, social support, lifestyle changes, and many prescription medicines are available. Unfortunately, there are situations when drug side effects can be hard to bear. Medication can be a viable solution or a short-term reaction to symptoms.

Anyone in a depressed state of mind needs a lasting solution. This needs time to recover from depression. Most people have turned to meditation, fitness, and other treatments for depression to better alleviate the symptoms. Yoga has been known to be a soft, active way to remove many of the depression symptoms.

Yoga is a way of connecting with one's selves. This helps people to go beyond everyday life thoughts and behaviors to concentrate on a larger purpose. Depressed people may continue to communicate with an internal sense of peace and relaxation through mindfulness, contemplation, careful breathing, relaxing, and strengthening. While any yoga practice will give about internal confidence and calmness, there are unique poses that will further cultivate it.

Child's Pose. This pose will bring great comfort and safety as the name implies. When students curl up close to a fetal position and put their foreheads on the floor, the stance bases the body and produces happy feelings.

Forward Bend. This posture triggers a great deal of the blood flowing out from the upper body, promoting contemplative thinking. Students also feel refreshed and energized as students break the posture and bring fresh blood supply flowing down the body.

Legs up the Wall. Legs taking the Wall posture down the bloodstream from the feet and legs to the middle of the body, providing a rooted look. This takes learners back to the present moment, helping them to unlock the past and the future and expose themselves to the now. Those with depression may begin to understand how necessary it is to release the fear and concentrate on a relaxed appearance. The movement to the limbs is restored as the posture is inverted.

This stretch requires students to concentrate on each motion on deep breathing. This helps students learn to consciously relax, and helps to relieve fear, uncertainty, and restlessness feelings.

Camel and Bridge. The back bent postures community exposes the whole body's neck and heart region. An open heart can, in figurative words, welcome new, positive experiences and expel existing, negative energy. It allows stressed students to unleash negative emotions that may have been holding in the core for a long time by actually doing the pose.

CONCLUSION

Depression can be a manageable challenge. A lot of help is available, and people have come before you and it. Start helping yourself by sending yourself a message that is a great builder of trust. Small successes can result in larger successes. It is a gradual process.

New therapies to fight depression are regularly discovered. Researchers make great progress in the treatment of depression. Although some are currently considered experimental or not approved by the FDA-Federal Drug Administration, some hospitals and clinics are offering transcranial magnetic stimulation in the case of TMS.

New drugs have fewer side effects and are better tolerated. Together, you and your doctor can decide the best treatment course for your specific needs.

We found a purely natural supplement to depression that can also help with anxiety and overall well-being.

You can use exercise and controlled dieting to ease your depression. Ask your doctor, find a nutritionist, read a book, and take action. Explore and start the possibilities of what's at your disposal. It is a healthy strategy to do something positive for yourself. Start today!

It is important to know what type of depression one is dealing with in the treatment of depression; as well as taking into account possible contributing factors, age, and typical developmental stage a person may be before taking the next step.

Licensed counselors, psychologists, and psychiatrists are all skilled in making a diagnosis of mental health. If the patient is a child or an elderly person, a person specializing in those developmental stages should complete the evaluation. Typically, counselors are equipped to provide people with depression with therapeutic guidance.

One can learn new ways of seeing their problems in counseling, develop enhanced coping skills, and find relief in having some external supports. Psychologists generally provide tests and evaluations that can determine the types and severity of mental health problems more accurately. Psychologists may prescribe medicines in some states and provide advice.

Psychiatrists seldom provide advice. Their role is to medically treat symptoms of mental health-usually with psychotropic drugs. Increasing physical activity and improving nutritional health is a general rule of thumb in the treatment of all forms of mental health issues. There are also numerous alternative treatments, including acupuncture, amino acid / nutritional therapies, mediation, energy work such as Reiki, EFT, bodywork, and N.E. T. (Neuro-Emotional Technique).

There is help if you, or someone you know, are experiencing persistent or severe symptoms of depression. Consider obtaining an evaluation of mental health and exclude any possible medical causes. Untreated depression can lead to long-term problems with health, substance abuse, and a lifetime of pain.

Help is available and depression can be 100% curable!

CPSIA information can be obtained
at www.ICGtesting.com
Printed in the USA
LVHW050817220221
679596LV00032B/2074